The Medicine Man among the Zaramo of Dar es Salaam

The Medicine Man

among the Zaramo of Dar es Salaam

Lloyd Swantz

Published by
the Scandinavian Institute of African Studies in cooperation with
Dar es Salaam University Press

Cover: Zaramo Mganga Ndamba, photo by Ingmar Lindqvist

Editing: Mai Palmberg

Type-setting: English Unlimited Ltd
Esbo 02230 Finland

ISBN 91-7106-299-8

Printed in Sweden by
Bohusläningen, Uddevalla 1990

CONTENTS

INTRODUCTION

This book is based on my Doctoral Thesis "The role of the medicine man among the Zaramo of Dar es Salaam" presented at the University of Dar es Salaam in 1974. The original study began as an attempt to understand the urban Zaramo and the forces which work to preserve their traditional values and culture as well as help them to adjust to the new urban situations. Quite unexpectedly, the *mganga*, the medicine man, emerged as the one member of society who was involved with most areas of Zaramo life. To find the answers to my questions I was compelled to concentrate my attention on the role of the *mganga* amongst the Zaramo. This edited version of the thesis omits the basic ethnographic descriptive material given in the original, which covered in detail the history, religious beliefs, social structure of the Zaramo, and examined present day urban-rural interrelationships among them.

Over the past one hundred years the medicine man and his work has been grossly misrepresented and misunderstood. Western sensationalism has attached to him the name "Witch-doctor", which calls up visions of bizarre stereotypes of Africans which are both inaccurate and offensive. Rather than generalizations and assumptions of what many people think medicine men are and do, in-depth investigations are needed. Reliable, representative and empirical data needed to be collected on which we could objectively and sympathetically analyze what actually is being done by African traditional healers. This study is an attempt to do just that. Furthermore, it was done in the setting of an African city, Dar es Salaam, the capital of independent Tanzania. This is not a history of past practices but places the medicine man in the context of modern urban society with all its hopes for development, modernization and social change.

It was my hope that by interviewing and analyzing the work of numerous medicine men and their clients, we might arrive at a more accurate understanding of this traditional healing profession which touches the lives of innumerable Africans, as indeed of people on all continents.

It was not within my competence, nor in the nature of the material, to determine how successful the medicine man or woman is as a medical practitioner. There is no scientific medical way at present to measure the results of their medicine and therapy. We can measure only what they claim to do and what problems people refer to them, as well as the clients' evaluation of their treatment. This is a study of opinions, beliefs and reported activity, not a scientific analysis of traditional medicine and its therapeutic results.

The Zaramo people constitute the largest single ethnic group living in Dar es Salaam. Not only are they numerically the largest urban body of

Tanzania, but they represent similar ethnic groups of peoples from the coastal area which make up fully one half of the total population of Dar es Salaam.

To know the Zaramo is to know what goes on in the lives of half the population of the city. At the time of the 1967 census, there were 19,122 Zaramo households in Dar es Salaam which would mean about 63,000 people. To this figure could be added several thousands more who live on the periphery of the city and thus are not included in the census.

I chose three representative areas of the city from which to administer questionnaires to 150 Zaramo: Ilala-Buguruni, Kariakoo and Magomeni. The sample of informants was selected by visiting every fifth house on the street or in the area. An equal number of men and women were interviewed. These 150 Zaramo informants were adherents to Islam: ninety-eight per cent of the Zaramo population are Muslim, and only 2 per cent are Christian.

One hundred Zaramo clients of *waganga* were interviewed mainly in the waiting rooms of the *waganga's* premises and, thus, also represented a fair cross-section of the Zaramo population living in various parts of the city. As waiting for the *mganga* often involved sitting for a number of hours, it meant that information from the clients could be gathered in a natural, unrushed manner.

In order to locate practising medicine men, a street-by-street search was made in the Ilala and Kariakoo ("Mission Quarter") areas. A total of 53 traditional medicine men and 7 Muslim clerics practising medicine were found and interviewed in these two areas. An additional 30 medicine men and 2 Muslim cleric practitioners were interviewed in other major areas of the city.

At first it was thought that *waganga* would be suspicious and unco-operative with strangers and in particular with a European seeking information about their work. For the most part this proved not to be so, but it was usually a very slow process to get to meet them during their working hours. The procedure was to sit in line with the other clients waiting to see the *mganga* for treatment. Because of the hours of waiting involved, usually no more than two *waganga* could be interviewed in a day.

We approached the *waganga* unannounced, like any other patient. Then we stated simply that we were from the University College of Dar es Salaam and were writing a book about the work of the *waganga* in the city. We asked if they would have a few minutes to give us a little information and whether we could return at a more convenient time for additional information. The response, with few exceptions, was positive and open. On a number of visits we were allowed to observe the *mganga* as he dealt with his patients. Through revisits and after gaining the confidence of several *waganga* to the point of becoming friends, we were able to obtain the information needed for this study.

I think that it was actually an advantage to me to have been a non-African in this context, because there could be no fear on their part that I might have been collecting free information in order to become a *mganga* myself, nor that I might sell the information or use it against them. Although not always fully understanding the reason for the research, most informants seemed pleased when told that the information would be put into a book which their children could one day read. The *waganga* did not try to hide the fact that they were practising traditional or Islamic medicine, which indicated that they did not sense any conflict between their work and the general government policies. Neither did it appear that they practised socially unacceptable medicine, even though some such aspects would seem inherent in their work.

Three basic methods were used in gathering information over a period of five years: (1) questionnaires, (2) interviews, and (3) observations. The findings were constantly compared with the rural Zaramo research which was being conducted at the same time by my wife, Marja-Liisa Swantz.

Although the questionnaires provided invaluable information concerning the knowledge, attitudes and practices of the Zaramo, this study is not based primarily on questionnaires. They were used mainly as an introduction to the various topics and to gain some quantitative data about the changes taking place in thought and practice. Deeper insight and additional inside information was gained through discussions and interviews. The results of the questionnaires were then either verified or shown to be misleading. In addition to interviews with 84 *waganga*, 9 Muslim clerics, 100 clients and the Zaramo general survey, I had additional interviews and tape recorded conversations with no fewer than 200 further Zaramo informants.

I was fortunate in having Mr. Ajuaye Chuma as a full-time research assistant for three years. He is a Zaramo school teacher and an experienced interviewer, fluent in both Swahili and Zaramo. He administered the questionnaires and conducted the interviews in close consultation with me, and he also did extensive translation of Zaramo and Swahili texts and tape recordings into English. I do not believe that the quality of information gained by him could have been obtained as accurately or quickly by a European or non-Zaramo Tanzanian interviewer. A second Zaramo, Mr. Levi Sozigwa, was employed in 1970 for several months to gather and discuss additional information on Zaramo customs and the work of *waganga* and to check the material previously collected.

I am grateful to Dr. Stephen Lucas who was my advisor, to my wife Marja-Liisa Swantz and to all others who supported and encouraged me in this research.

Lloyd W. Swantz
Helsinki January 1989

Terminology

In this study I use the Swahili word *mganga* interchangeably with its English equivalent, medicine man (*Waganga* designates the plural). These two words will not hereafter be italicized in the text simply on the grounds of their frequent use in the book. Non-English words will normally be designated as Zaramo, Swahili or other. If no designation follows the word, it may be assumed to be a Swahili word. A glossary of terms is given at the end of the book.

Abbreviations

Ar. = Arabic

L. = Latin

Lu. = Luguru

Lit. = Literal translation

Pl. = Plural

S. = Singular

Sw. = Swahili

Z. = Zaramo

CHAPTER 1
Traditional Medicine Men and Muslim Clerics as Healers

A new arrival walking through the streets of residential Dar es Salaam would not detect that here and there on almost every street there are full-time practitioners of traditional medicine at work. There are no signs or markings on the houses to indicate their presence. The houses in which the traditional healers conduct their practice appear identical to other residential houses in the area. Most of the homes in the older residential areas are built according to the Swahili type of architecture with wattle filled in with mud and plastered over with cement. In the redevelopment housing areas the same style is constructed with cement blocks and corrugated iron or aluminium roof sheeting. People slip practically unnoticed through the doorway of such an inconspicuous home to seek help from the mganga, medicine man or woman, located there.

Dar es Salaam residents seeking medical aid may visit a traditional mganga located in the housing areas, but there are also other medical practitioners or dispensers of medicine to whom they might turn. This study is primarily concerned with the traditional mganga, but in order to gain a more complete picture, other specialists are also considered briefly. They are the Muslim sheikhs and Koran teachers in the role of mganga, the herbalists, the itinerant witchcraft eradicators, the shrine keepers, the street sellers and the traditional circumcisers and midwives. Some of these are not considered waganga nor are they addressed as waganga, but they dispense medicine or perform a medical function.

1. The Traditional Waganga

The term "traditional mganga" is used here to describe a person who practises healing after the pattern of the traditional art of medicine and healing within his or her ethnic group. There are many Dar es Salaam people who have some knowledge of herbs and roots which are effective against certain illnesses and use them in their own family for curing. These people are not considered here as waganga. Waganga sell their services to others on a business basis. "Traditional" does not mean that there is any one static form of tribal medical practice nor that waganga follow only the forms of medicine of their own ethnic group. The traditional medicine man has most often learned from others within the same tribe, but a considerable number have learned their *uganga,* medicine or medical treatment, from men or women of other ethnic groups. It is often believed that the *uganga* of another tribe is more powerful.

The term "traditional waganga" is thus used here for the men and women who practise their healing art for the public and do so primarily in the manner carried out by the waganga of their tribe in rural areas. There have been changes and adaptations, but in general their methods adhere closely to the manner in which healing was practised before Western medicine and Islamic forms of healing were introduced.

The traditional mganga is not prohibited from practising his or her system of therapeutics under Tanzanian law. The country still operates under laws constituted before Independence which remain largely the same today. Cap. 92.20 contains the *Medical Practitioners and Dentists Ordinance*, which reads:

> Nothing contained in this ordinance shall be construed to prohibit or prevent the practise of systems of therapeutics according to native methods by persons recognized by the community to which they belong to be duly trained in such practice.
>
> Provided that nothing in this section shall be construed to authorize any person to practise native systems of therapeutics except amongst the community to which he belongs, or the performance of an act on the part of any persons practising any such system which is dangerous to life.[1]

This law seems to be designed for a rural community where the people of a particular tribe would know the mganga to be "duly trained" and would accept the practice of that mganga. The law speaks of the mganga practising "amongst the community to which he belongs." To which community does an urban mganga belong? In a detribalized urban community the waganga are not recognized by a "community" but only by the individuals who seek their aid. Their practise does not operate on tribal lines which indeed today would be out of harmony with the country and the law. What community then is responsible for legitimating or "recognizing" the practice of an urban mganga? This we must leave for the lawyers to work out. In the meantime, the waganga continue their practise unmolested, unchallenged and at peace with the law and the community.

In the absence of any directory of waganga in Dar es Salaam or of signboards identifying their place of practice, they can be found only through the recommendation of other persons who know their location. In Dar es Salaam the most common way to find a mganga is to ask a friend to recommend a "good one." The average person normally will know of several waganga and can supply their addresses. Some waganga have a good reputation for treating certain types of problems such as dizziness, epilepsy, stomach disorders, mental illness and sorcery-related misfortunes.

A friend generally recommends the mganga who is reputed to be adept at curing the particular problem at hand. A second method, which was used in this study to locate medicine men in a specific area of the city, was simply to walk down a street and ask people every few houses if any waganga were living in the immediate area. This method was tried in the Ilala area and in one section of Kariakoo, the "Mission Quarter" area.

There is no easy way to determine the total number of full-time medicine men practising in Dar es Salaam. It is puzzling that no traditional practitioners were reported in the occupation survey made by J. Leslie in his *Social Survey of Dar es Salaam* in 1957 or in the occupational survey included in the Marco Survey study of Dar es Salaam conducted for the government in 1964-65. I checked hundreds of the 1967 census returns from the Ilala and Kariakoo section of my study area, and found that not one head of household who completed the questionnaire listed himself as a mganga. It is my contention that medicine men do not wish to be publicly known for fear that someone in the government might check on their income tax payments. Waganga, including Muslim *washehe* and *walimu* who practise forms of healing, may be among the highest-paid Tanzanians in Dar es Salaam and therefore reticent lest their lucrative practice be brought to the attention of the revenue officers.

In the sector of Ilala where every street was canvassed for medicine men, 39 were found plus an additional 4 Muslim *walimu* and one *shehe* who practised healing. Dividing the known total of 44 practitioners among the approximate 20,000 people living in the area, amounts to one mganga for every 454 people. It is likely that several more *washehe* and *walimu* should be added to this list, and some waganga could also have been missed. In the "Mission Quarter" area of Kariakoo, where approximately 5,000 people live, 11 waganga, two *washehe* and one *mwalimu* were located. This would average out to one medical practitioner for every 375 people. This means that if one accepts the 1968 figure of 250,000 Africans living in Dar es Salaam then there are 700 practising medicine men in the city. This number does not include the itinerant medicine men, the herb street sellers, the bottled medicine street hawkers or *muwizi*, circumcisers.

In the questionnaire which was administered to 150 Zaramo, the question of occupation was asked. According to this survey, there were three full-time traditional healers for 150 adult Zaramo. If this ratio was carried over into the total adult Zaramo population in Dar es Salaam, it would again mean that there were approximately 700 Zaramo medicine men in Dar es Salaam, not counting the Muslim Koran teachers and *washehe*.[2] This confirms the street-by-street survey.

The sample may be somewhat small to draw any definite numerical conclusions; but when it is compared with the rural studies of M-L Swantz, who found the ratio for the rural village of Bunju to be 4:100, we see the ratio of waganga to the population to be much the same. Her figures are based on actual waganga interviewed, but there were undoubtedly others in the community who were missed. Therefore, on the basis of actual interviews with known medicine men in Dar es Salaam; estimates from a sample of 150 Zaramo Muslim adults; plus a comparison with a rural Zaramo ratio, we can conservatively estimate that there were no fewer than 700 full-time traditional medical practitioners working in Dar es Salaam in the early 1970s, and that more than likely the number in reality was considerably larger. In fact, it is one of the larger occupational groupings in the city, even though it fails to appear on occupational surveys.

The largest number of medicine men in Dar es Salaam were Zaramo. They number 51, representing 61 per cent of the group interviewed. The second largest group were Rufiji (6), 9.5 per cent, and the third largest the Kwere (5), 6 per cent. Twelve ethnic groups were represented amongst the waganga. The only major inland tribe represented was the Nyamwezi with four waganga.

The waganga were asked which ethnic groups of people they treated. The Zaramo were listed first in almost every answer, even though the mganga may have been of a different ethnic group. Waganga do not treat only those of their own ethnic group, but take clients from all tribes. It is natural that the Zaramo, who are the majority ethnic group in the city, would also have the greatest number of both waganga and clients. The Zigua, Hehe, Yao and Arabs were also occasionally listed as clients. In none of the interviews with medicine men and their clients did I detect any feeling of tribal prejudice. Nor did I find any tribal or professional jealousy or animosity among the waganga themselves.

2. The Call and Training of the Mganga

What is the motivation which leads men and women in this present age to become practitioners of traditional medicine when they must be aware that the trend in modern society is towards "scientific" medicine? Is it just a matter of time and a little more education and then all the waganga will go out of business?

At the beginning of the 1970s there was a shortage of Tanzanians trained in "scientific" medicine. Of the some 200 registered government doctors in Dar es Salaam, not more than a quarter were Tanzanians and not one was Zaramo. What then called the estimated 700 traditional medicine men to go into full-time business in Dar es Salaam, outnumbering the government and private doctors at least three to one and asking for no government subsidy or favours?

Fifty-six medicine men were asked how they became waganga. The answers given were not always as clear as desired, and one could surmise from the *uganga* practised that they may have had more than one type of training. The information given suggest seven distinct patterns by which a person might acquire *uganga* today.

TABLE 1: Responses to the Question: How did you get your *Uganga* ?

Response	No. [Respondents]
I was taught (apprenticeship) by my father, grandfather or unrelated mganga	10
I inherited the *mfuko* (medicine bag), and was taught	11
I had Islamic training in *uganga*	21
I had Islamic training in *uganga* and also studied under a mganga	5
I inherited a *mzimu* spirit and *uganga*	3
I was possessed by the spirit and had to take up *uganga* or remain ill	3
I just picked up the knowledge *hivi hivi* from here and there	3
TOTAL	56

In addition to the above 56 waganga, it can be assumed that the three *washehe*, Muslim clerics, and six *walimu*, Koran teachers, had all undergone Islamic training in geomancy and other *elimu ya dunia* , education of the world, either in the more organized schools at Bagamoyo, Kilwa or Zanzibar, or under the direction of another *shehe* or *mwalimu* . Of the nine

Muslim clerics and teachers, four also healed using herbs as well as the *Kitabu*, Book. This would indicate that they might also have studied under a traditional mganga or acquired knowledge from another Muslim mganga versed in traditional medicine.

Of the 21 traditional waganga who used Islamic forms of healing, 17 indicated that they also used herbs and the traditional *uganga* methods. This indicates that they may have studied under a traditional mganga as well as having the Islamic training.

Ten waganga said they were taught and eleven said they inherited the *mfuko*, medicine bag, from other waganga after they had died. A few examples from case records will illustrate this:

> Mganga M. started learning *uganga* in childhood while his father was alive. "My father taught me how to play the rattles (*Rungu* divining) (see Chapter 3) and sing when I was about ten years old. I was singing with him when he made *ramli* divining. When I became older I became his *kizumilo*, helper. My father also played *madogoli kupunga mashetani*, exorcised spirits through *madogoli* rites, so that I also learned this. All my *uganga* is from my father. I have inherited it. I can make *ramli*, divine, treat sickness and *kupunga madogoli*. My father taught and showed me many different kinds of medicines and trees I know myself. I know many kinds of medicines. I am not trying to be proud, but I know my dead parents, *wahenga*, and God helps me."[3]

It is well to note that mganga could speak about learning his *uganga* from his father or inheriting it from his father. This is why the 11 who answered " I inherited the *mfuko* and was taught" may be more accurately reported than the ten who simply stated "I was taught... " It is possible that most of these were being taught under an apprenticeship system and had no relationship to the instructing mganga, but the possibility cannot be excluded that a number of them, as in the group of 11, had also inherited their *uganga.*

If a parent is a mganga, one of the children, either male or female, will invariably inherit the medicine bag. Before or after the official receiving of the medicine bag there is some form of instruction or apprenticeship. The apprentice training period may last from a few months to many years, depending on the age of the trainee when he or she starts.

Mganga M. stated that he had started training as a boy of ten years and studied under his father until he was about 20 years old. There is no official "graduating" exercise or examination. It is up to the senior mganga to determine whether or not the apprentice has sufficient knowledge and experience to work alone. When this happens the mganga will announce this to the other waganga of the community, who then treat the former apprentice as an equal. If he or she is a mganga of one of the spirits there will be invitations to take part in some of the public rites, and soon the word gets around that the new mganga is fully qualified and can take clients of his or her own.

In the city, this system of apprenticeship and approval by the neighboring waganga and community may break down. If a mganga moves into the city from the country, who is to know whether or not he or she had any training and is considered qualified by other waganga? There is no certificate needed or medical board to consider their qualifications and training. As indicated in the answers given regarding training, three said they had just picked up the knowledge "*hivi hivi*", here and there. Of the 17 who said they had inherited the medicine bag, we do not know how they acquired their knowledge of *uganga*. It may also have been "*hivi hivi* ". To begin their practice, waganga need only a few friends to recommend them to others and a reasonable amount of success in their practice so that their first clients will also recommend them to others.

Mganga M. said that he had several men studying *uganga* under him. He spoke of his pupils in this manner: "I have some pupils at home. Some on the *madogoli* and some on *ramli* . They are OK. I trust them. They can go anywhere and they will never get any troubles." By this he meant that they now had the knowledge to counter sorcery and would not be overcome by the power of those practising sorcery.

About half of the waganga interviewed in Dar es Salaam had such students or what they sometimes called *wasaidizi*, helpers. These are usually younger men or boys who are training on the job. They help prepare the medicines and stand by the mganga as he heals the clients, bringing the mganga whatever roots, herbs or materials he requests. Some said they use their helpers to collect medicine from the forest and countryside. The apprentices learn the trade by observing; there are no books to read on the non-Islamic forms of *uganga*. The tuition paid for such on-the-job training varies from one hundred to two hundred shillings, depending on the length of training and the age of the student. Part of the fee is paid at the beginning of the training and the remainder at the end. The mganga however receives free labor for several years from his student, and this must be considered part of the agreement.

The largest group of the waganga had some form of Islamic *uganga* and divining. As children they might have spent several years at Koranic school, where they began to learn Arabic and memorized portions of the Koran. If they wished to become Muslim clerics or to learn Islamic forms of *uganga* they would study privately under a *shehe* or *mwalimu*. Some study under medicine men using Islamic forms of *ramli* and *uganga* but who are not practising Muslim clerics. This form of education includes the study of *elimu ya dunia*, lit. "education of the world", but centers on the art of Islamic healing and divining. Students learn various *sura*, chapters from the Koran and other Islamic writings, which are considered to be efficacious incantations for healing, protecting, cursing and counter-sorcery power. The names of angels and *jini* must be known as well as the power and value system connected with numbers, symbols, times and seasons of the year.

The *Satrikhabari* seems to be the most commonly studied and widely used book for Islamic forms of healing and divining. Other books studied and used in the East African coastal area, according to Trimingham, are the treatise of Muhammad az-Zanati, *Kitab al-fasl fi usul ar-raml* and *Ta'bir ar-ru'ya* by Ibn Sirin (Trimingham, 1964, 124). Verses from the book *Hal Badiri*, Ar., *Halubadili*, Sw., must be known, as this is one of the main readings for cursing others and for protection. Islamic words and phrases must be memorized as well as chapters and verses from the Koran. These are written in Arabic by the mganga and put into protection amulets, good luck charms, and used in healing.

The training in the Islamic *uganga* may also continue for several years, depending on the age and memory capacity of the pupil. This training includes reading and memory work as well as observing and helping the *shehe*, *mwalimu* or mganga in his practice. The student pays the teacher for this tuition much the same as others pay a mganga for tutoring and on-the-job experience. Some of these pupils may be interested only in learning Islamic *uganga*, but others train to be *mwalimu* and Muslim clerics. Five of the 56 waganga questioned said they had received Islamic training as well as training from the traditional mganga, whereas 21 of the 56 said they had received only Islamic training in *uganga*. The latter was the largest single group and indicates the strong Islamic influence in the practice of *uganga* in Dar es Salaam.

Three of the waganga interviewed stated that they had inherited a *mzimu*, spirit shrine, and its accompanying *uganga* (see Chapter 2). All three spirit huts or shrines were located at the foot of large baobab trees in Dar es Salaam. These waganga inherited the *mzimu* from their fathers who were waganga and keepers of the *mzimu* before them. They speak of themselves as "owners" of the *mzimu* and collect accordingly the money left by people using the *mzimu*. Very little training would be necessary to own a *mzimu* spirit shrine hut, but as the three waganga were all practising medicine in addition to this responsibility, they would have had some training in *uganga* from their fathers or others.

Three waganga stated that they had been possessed by a spirit and therefore were compelled to take up the practice of *uganga* to avoid continued illness or death. Mganga M. stated: "My grandfather was a mganga, but during his lifetime I neglected it. After my grandfather died I fell sick. The diviner told me to go home and take my grandfather's medicine bag. That's how I got it. I was foolish to neglect it. Now I am living happily because of it. "

Mganga A.S. suffered mental illness for two years. His relatives consulted three different waganga, but he was not cured. Finally it was revealed to him by a spirit that he was being troubled by the Rungu spirit. After being exorcized and initiated into the Rungu spirit cult he became well. "From that time on I had to do this work. I do not like it, but I got my health back because of it."

An additional three waganga said they just picked up their knowledge of *uganga* "hivi hivi", here and there. "I got *uganga* by being very clever," said one. "I picked it up from different people," said another. This I believe may be the case also with many others who did not wish to offer information on how they acquired their *uganga.* Perhaps they had no formal training but were good observers and had gradually worked themselves into business. We do not have substantial statistics on the number of inactive waganga in the city. Since most of the waganga, like the rest of the population, have come to the city from the rural areas, it is very likely that they return to the countryside if they are not successful. There is no way to count these returnees. An indication that there are a considerable number of inactive waganga in the city arises from the occupational question in my general survey of 150 Zaramo. In this survey I found three practising waganga amongst 75 men and two others who had inherited the medicine bag but were not practising. Amongst the 75 Zaramo women there were two waganga and three others who held the medicine bag but did not practise. These figures suggest that perhaps as many as one-half of the Zaramo who would be entitled by inheritance rights to practise *uganga* do not do so. I have no information as to whether they were trained and failed or whether they had the bag but were not interested in going into the practice.

In the actual street-by-street survey of the Ilala area we found no practising women waganga. From rural studies we know that there are women waganga and we know from the 150 Zaramo Survey that some women have the medicine bag and say they are waganga. But, when the street-by-street search was made they were not found. It would appear that women are not accepted as waganga to the same degree in urban Muslim society as in the rural Zaramo society, where Islam exists side by side with *Pazi* traditional religion. It may very well be that Muslim social pressure hinders women waganga from practising and that they constitute the largest number of those who leave the profession.

The age range of the traditional medicine men fell between 30 and 65 years, with 42 years being the average age. The *uganga* practitioners amongst the Muslim *shehe* and *mwalimu* ranged from 40 to 70 years, with 56 being the average age. The helpers and men in training were between the ages of 16 and 30 years. There may be several reasons why the age level of the Muslim *shehe* and *mwalimu* is higher than the traditional waganga. The calling of a *shehe* and *mwalimu* is usually a life time occupation continuing until death. African mosques in Dar es Salaam, in contrast to mosques used by Indians and Arabs, are owned by the *shehe* himself. The mosque passes from father to son through inheritance. Because this inheritance depends on death and not retirement, it raises the age level of the group considerably. Also, fewer young men are going into the Muslim cleric and teaching profession because with the public education offered by the government, the number of Koran pupils is decreasing and the time of study shortened, thus offering fewer jobs for Koranic teachers.

The average length of practise for waganga in the Ilala, Buguruni and Kariakoo areas was 15 $^1/_2$ years. A number of the waganga had practised in villages before coming to Dar es Salaam. If a similar sample were taken in Magomeni, Mansese and Kinondoni, the years of practise would be less, for these are newer housing areas. It is quite likely that anyone wishing to go into business today would settle in the rapidly expanding areas on the outer edge of the city. It is here that the newly arriving Zaramo find housing and it is amongst these people who are already familiar with the practice of *uganga* from their home villages, that the waganga will find his best customers.

It may be asked: By what authority and process of legitimization do the traditional practitioners assume their role in the urban society? The rural mganga's role is still mainly legitimized through inheritance and often accompanied by charismatic experiences which play an important part (Swantz, M-L, 1970, 394-399). For the rural mganga, the practice is not mainly for monetary gain. Even in cases where the mganga has inherited the practice, he or she has usually assumed it under an inner compulsion or has had a spirit experience which has laid the obligation on them.

We have seen in the material the legitimization of the mganga's role first by the right of inheritance. Refusal of the *mfuko*, medicine bag, when in line for it by inheritance, would be a sign of great disrespect. To neglect it, the Zaramo believe, would most certainly result in illness or misfortune for that individual. Likewise, a spirit shrine, *mzimu*, is acquired by inheritance, and the new owner is likely, though not always, to be instructed in *uganga*.

Second, there is an assuming of the mganga's position after a period of apprenticeship under another mganga. Many of those who inherit the profession from their father or grandfather also study under them or assist them for many years. Others study under another mganga or a Muslim cleric even after officially receiving the medicine bag.

Some of the interviewed waganga said they found their authority to practise *uganga* in the event of spirit possession, thus being forced to take up the practice by that spirit. Others say they received their "call" in a dream or in a trance-like state where they believed they were taken to the top of a tall tree or to the bottom of a lake and kept there until they promised to become waganga. Such accounts are never doubted by the general Zaramo public, and thereafter the person is considered a bona fide mganga. Similar dream and trance-like "calls" to the *uganga* profession are found in many parts of Africa and are considered just as legitimate as receiving the profession by inheritance or apprenticeship. To ignore such a "call" by a spirit is thought to result in serious illness or even death.

In Dar es Salaam there is no easy way to check on how a person has acquired his or her *uganga*. It would be possible for anybody to move into the city from the country and, being unknown to the population, establish himself as a mganga. Three out of the 56 waganga interviewed on this question admitted that they just picked up their knowledge of *uganga "hivi hivi"*, here and there.

Only three respondents out of 56 waganga said they practised because of what could be called a charismatic experience through spirit possession. All the others had inherited the *uganga* or had received it through an apprenticeship or training. However the majority of urban waganga keep at their occupation only as long as people come to them and are willing to pay the high fees.

The real test of the profession comes in the skill and ability of the waganga, whatever the manner of their entry into the practise. If they are successful in their therapeutic method and if they can assure the client of their power to protect or their ability to discern a situation, their role as waganga is secure.

The vast majority of Zaramo do not question the waganga's authority to practise. Their calling is not doubted. They are an accepted institution in Zaramo society and are considered as workers of good. During the research for this study it was rare to hear adverse comments about waganga from the people interviewed. No mganga doubted or criticized the work or authority of another mganga. For the present, public opinion, tradition and demand assures the successful mganga a place in Zaramo urban society.

3. The Urban Mganga's Consulting Room

The medicine man's consulting room in Dar es Salaam is not noticeable to the stranger passing by on the street. There is no sign or symbol to indicate services of the waganga. Until 1970 there was not a single mganga sign in the whole of Dar es Salaam. Then one day in mid-1970 a new Swahili-type house was built in Kigogo with a notice board outside, and even one on a nearby corner, announcing the new practice of a medicine man. To my knowledge this was the first to appear in the city.[4] All other waganga must be found by enquiry, mainly through the recommendation and direction of a friend. If the mganga has a good reputation, clients will readily travel great distances to seek his or her help. There are a number of waganga in the city whose reputation is widely known and whose daily case load is several times larger than that of the average mganga.

The majority of waganga in the sample owned their own homes, and about a quarter of them owned two or more houses in Dar es Salaam. These were usually the Swahili-type houses with six rooms, a courtyard in the back and a few outer rooms for the latrine, washroom and extra sleeping rooms. The clients wait outside in the rear courtyard until their turns come to enter the mganga's consultation room. They sit on benches, chairs or mats on the ground. During the rainy season they may sit on benches in the central passage way of the house. Most waganga have only one room for meeting their clients. A few will have an adjoining second room for storing roots and bottles and where the helper or apprentice sleeps. Depending on the number of wives and children he has, a mganga will use one or two additional rooms in the house as his living quarters, renting out the others.

A number of waganga who treated mental patients had one or two rooms in the house or in the outer courtyard where such patients could be kept for short periods as in-patients. The mental patients could thus be treated several times a day and return to their rooms. Relatives stayed in the rooms with such patients to care for them. I am not aware of any other type of illness for which in-patient care was given.

The clients may sometimes use the washroom in the rear of the courtyard for bathing with the medicines given to them by the mganga. There is seldom running water or a shower in the washroom, so the client is provided with a pail of water in which to put his medicine for washing.

The mganga's office is usually one room, plainly furnished and not unlike other rooms in a Swahili-type house. In the cases observed, on almost every occasion the clients were asked to remove their shoes before entering the mganga's room. Plain mats cover the floor. In most cases the mganga sits on a pillow or stool in the middle of the floor and the client sits on the mat or stool before him. If a chair, table or bench is in the room it is against the wall. The tables are usually piled high with bottles, gourds, roots and leaves.

Scattered around the mganga where he sits on the floor are his divining materials such as the *bao*, divining board, rattles or books, which he might consult. This depends on what type of divining he uses (see Chapter 3). Also beside him usually is a supply of herbs, roots, papers, a slate, a Koran and whatever types of medicines he uses for his *uganga*. If the mganga is one of a particular spirit he normally has beside him his *mfuko*, medicine bag, in which he keeps his gourd of medicine and an assortment of red, white and black cloth used in the treatments. A wildebeest tail whisk and the traditional axe might also be lying about, as they are the insignia for most waganga, but are seldom used other than in *ngomas* performed at outdoor exorcism rites.

If what the mganga needs for the treatment is not immediately available, he might call his helper to fetch what is needed. In some cases the client has been asked at a previous consultation to bring along a chicken, cloth and particular ingredients for some medicines. Also on the floor nearby is a round charcoal stove on which is an aluminium or clay pot filled with boiling water kept ready for use. Cold water is stored in a large clay pot resting on an iron frame or else in pails along the side of the wall. Some consultation rooms in the city central areas have electric lights, but most others, particularly in Buguruni, Kigogo and Kawe areas, use paraffin lamps.

The consulting room of the *shehe* or *mwalimu* do not differ greatly from those of the traditional waganga. These practitioners do not treat their clients in the mosque or in the *baraza*, classroom, but rather in their homes which are often located near the mosque or in the house where the school is located. The only noticeable difference from the traditional waganga might be in the better quality of the furniture and dress. Also, because the Koran is the main method of treatment, herbs, roots and other medicines are not often seen in the rooms. A few *shehe* and *mwalimu* do use herbs together with the Koran, a factor which will be discussed at a later point.

Most waganga dress in a white *kanzu*, a Muslim type robe made from light cotton cloth. It extends to the floor over the underskirt and trousers. Some of the waganga wear a suit-coat over the *kanzu*, a style introduced into East Africa by the Sultan of Zanzibar in the late nineteenth century. The Arab-type embroidered cap is also commonly worn. A few waganga wear beads about the neck and arms, and underneath their clothing one may notice from time to time an amulet worn for protection. A few tie a red or yellow cloth sash around their waist during working hours.

Apart from the very few who wear a simple string of beads or a sash, most waganga are not discernible from other people walking down the street in their area. They tend to dress according to the current Muslim style rather than with a shirt and tie and European suit. On no occasion have waganga in Dar es Salaam been seen wearing furs, horns or the assortment of beads and regalia associated with waganga in other parts of Africa. In the rural areas, for the *madogoli* exorcism rites waganga are sometimes seen with a headdress and other equipment such as bells and beadwork. I have witnessed one *madogoli* performed in a rural area outside Dar es Salaam, when both the main mganga and the client had come from the city. The mganga wore a *colomba* monkey fur headdress, a number of beaded armbands and had bells fastened to both legs.

Apart from electric lights in some offices, no trend toward modernization can be observed in the medicine man's facilities. The positive side of this is that the clients feel immediately at home with the mganga. There is none of the strangeness that they encounter when going to the hospital or clinic. To my knowledge there is no attempt on the part of waganga to give injections or pharmaceutical medicines purchased at the chemist's shop. No attempt is made to examine the patients' bodily ailments, to take a blood test or to check the heart beat. Waganga never ask their patients to undress, for they make no physical examinations. I am not aware of any attempt at surgery, except for the small cuts occasionally made on the body for the purpose of rubbing in the medicine powder. The act of making incisions on the skin as part of the treatment appeared only once in the 100 cases observed. Because of the traditional type of medicine given, hygienic precautions such as washing and sterilization are not deemed necessary. As has been outlined here, the facilities needed to begin the work of *uganga* are very simple: a rented room in which to meet people, a mat, a stool, a stove and the knowledge of the profession.

4. The Mganga and His Patients

It is when we come to the mganga-patient relationship that we are touching an area where Western "scientific" medical practitioners would have a few points to learn from the traditional mganga. It is perhaps because of these personal relationships that the waganga are still so popular today and have a reputation for reasonable success.

First it must be said that the mganga has several factors in his favour even before he starts to work with his patient. The profession of *uganga* is a long-established and respected one in African traditional society. The mganga is looked upon with respect, if not with a little awe and wonder, because of his ability to divine and to know the secret things in life. He is considered a strong and powerful man of the spirit, for his ability rests not only in his medicine but in his *baraka*, a word which means blessing but is often used in this sense as the mganga's gift of inner powers. Therefore a client goes to a recommended mganga with considerable confidence that this man can help him.

In small villages people sometimes speak about their mganga as "my mganga" very much as people in America or Europe speak about their family doctor. Those people who have been possessed by a spirit and subsequently exorcised, from then on belong not only to that spirit but also to the mganga of the spirit. In this sense we speak of the spirit cult which people belong to and identify with (Swantz, M-L, 1970, 187 ff.). Because of this spirit cult relationship, many urban dwellers return to their particular mganga in the village for treatment of problems and for the *madogoli* exorcisms. In these client-mganga relationships each is known to the other and the mganga's business may be to keep himself well-informed about his client and all aspects of the village life.

In the city, with its large specialized hospitals and frequently rapid turnover of medical staff, often employing European doctors with little knowledge of the people or the language, the doctor-patient relationship is bound to be impersonal. Government medical clinics and hospitals in Dar es Salaam have thousands of out-patients each day, which means that a doctor may see his patient only once for a few brief minutes. He cannot possibly remember the patients' names, or even their faces, should they come a second time.

In the city many waganga are trying to build up a regular clientele, much as would be found in the village. Because of this personal relationship the Zaramo feel at home, and feel it is a continuation of an older cultural and social pattern known from their childhood in the country.

In the 150 Zaramo interviews the question was asked: "*Kwa mganga yupi wa kienyeji ambako huenda?* To which medicine man do you go for local medicine ?" Out of the 150 Zaramo informants, 30 % gave the name of their particular mganga. Of those 42 % were waganga located in Dar es Salaam and 58 % were from the countryside. This shows that even though people have moved away from the rural areas to the city over half of them still retain their home mganga relationship. Thirty percent keep the family mganga relationship, while 70 percent indicated that they consult various waganga but had chosen no particular one. Only six Zaramo mentioned that they go to their parents for home-brewed medicines. In other words, most Zaramo feel they need the professional service of a mganga and do not normally rely on their own or family remedies.

Although 58 per cent said their mganga was living in the country and gave the name of the mganga there, this may be misleading. It simply may have been easier to remember the name of an old well-established mganga used by their parents from childhood. If a person visits several different waganga in Dar es Salaam, he or she may not have been able to recall the name of any one person and therefore gave the name of the rural mganga. No question was asked as to the frequency of visits to the rural waganga. A person might feel a close relationship to an old mganga in the village but, because of the long distance, may go more often to the mganga in the city. Whatever the exact statistics may be, it does indicate that a strong relationship with the rural mganga exists, and we know from the rural studies that large numbers of urban Zaramo are found there on all ritual occasions.

Another factor in favour of going to the traditional mganga is that a Zaramo understands that his or her case will be considered more completely than would be possible at a government hospital. The mganga not only treats the illness or problem brought to him but can ascertain who caused it and for what reason. He can also offer protection so that it will not happen again. Western medicine can cure only certain types of illness, mainly of the body, while traditional practices are more comprehensive, dealing with the sickness caused by members of society or the spirit world as well as illness of the body. A Zaramo knows that the hospital cannot deal with sorcery, with angry or malevolent spirits, or with the "bad smell" which lingers after a prison term or which causes unemployment. The mganga takes into account religious and traditional beliefs as well as the social problems of the society. If people are under great stress because they believe themselves to be bewitched, no matter what medicine they are given at the hospital their state of tension will persist. A surprising number of informants who had first attended hospitals and did not regain their health said that they were told by the doctor to go home and try a medicine man. It is unlikely that European doctors would normally give such advice but there is no doubt that some medical assistants, nurses and attendants might recommend treatment by a mganga if they themselves were unsuccessful. So the Zaramo approaching a mganga knows he obtains the care of someone who believes and understands the complete problem. A European, Asian or African doctor with only Western medical training is not as equipped to handle the problem in a comprehensive manner.

The relationship between mganga and the client is a very cordial one. Each case is given individual attention and is followed through from the initial divining for the cause up to the provision of preventative protection medicine at the conclusion. Upon first contact, time is given for the exchange of greetings and the mganga is eager to learn as much as possible about his client. The mganga observes the client and in his divining may refer to some aspects of the client's behavior. He may observe general restlessness or fear and then speak about the troubled spirit of the patient. It seems obvious that the mganga has an intuitive capacity to gain insight into the client's character and life situation, although his success in this cannot be measured. If the mganga is unable to appraise his client satisfactorily, he may postpone the divining until another day, explaining that the stars are not clear so he cannot read the message. The mganga is motivated to serve and win a new client.

The briefest conversation with the mganga reveals the unquestioning confidence he has in his own *uganga* ability and that of other men and women in the profession. If you just mention the name of another mganga, he may go to great lengths to explain what a great *fundi*, craftsman, he is and what miracles he has performed. I have come to believe that waganga intentionally glorify each other's skill and practice in the eyes of the public, and that this mutual admiration has a positive effect on their corporate image. Everyone likes to repeat a good miracle healing story.

The mganga's confidence in his own *uganga* ability extends to the point where he is willing to take on any case or problem brought to him. When asked in interviews if they treat mental cases, some waganga answered, "I have had none yet, but I can try." It should be noted, however, that even though the mganga appears to boast of his abilities he will invariably conclude with a statement that he can succeed only "if God wills" or "if God helps."

The mutual trust in God's help and power, be it the faith of the Muslim, the Christian or the Pazi traditionalist, gives both mganga and client special confidence in what they are doing. It would be almost unthinkable for a mganga to deny belief in God and expect his clients to trust in his *uganga*. One story from a rural area illustrates the reaction of a client to a doctor who did not trust in God. In a Zaramo area of Ukutu, the Chinese, who were working on a railway project in the area, offered medical services to the local inhabitants. One Pazi traditional believer who was given medicine by the Chinese doctor expressed his gratefulness by saying , "*Mungu akujalie*, may God sustain you." To this the Chinese doctor replied, "Don't bring God into this; there is no God." The astonished Zaramo quickly handed back the medicine to the doctor and said, "Take your medicine back; if you don't believe in God this medicine can't be any good !" The traditional mganga is not ashamed of his belief in God. In at least half the treatments of Muslim and traditional practitioners some prayer or invocation to God is made. The fact that the Koran is used by so very many waganga in Dar es Salaam is evidence of this practice of invoking God's help.

In his work the mganga combines the roles of doctor and priest. He subscribes to the concept of the whole man, both the body and spirit, and recognizes that sin in the society and the guilt of his client or his enemy may be factors causing illness and misfortune. In some treatments a confession of guilt must be made before the mganga can proceed with the cure. A mganga once said to me after the client had left, "This person cannot be helped because she is the guilty one; she is getting what she deserves." If the mganga is unsuccessful in curing his patient, he can assume that his client is guilty of practising sorcery on someone who was protected and now the evil is coming back to her. The sin and guilt factor is taken into account as a mganga deals with the client.

Finally it can be said that the traditional waganga offer personalized medicine to their clients. They do not supply pills from a big bottle and write prescriptions to be taken to a stranger in a chemist's shop. Instead, the waganga make medicine specifically for the individual clients; it is personal medicine. The waganga normally go out into the bush to find the leaves or roots to make the particular medicine needed for their clients. In the city they may have a supply of leaves and herbs on hand. The client sees the medicine in the raw state and can watch the mganga compound it while he waits.

While the client sits before the charcoal stove the mganga drops the roots, leaves, coffee, needles or whatever the prescription calls for, into the pot of boiling water. If the mganga is using Islamic methods of curing, the client may watch him write in Arabic on the wooden *kombe*, board, after which water is poured over the wet ink and collected as a medical drink. Whatever is done, be it magical or authentic medicine making, clients have no doubt that they are getting proper attention and that the medicine is just for them.

If in the course of treatment a mganga does not gain the confidence of the patient by creating an atmosphere of concern and trust or by presenting the *uganga* in a way understandable to the client, he may fail in much of his effort. A rational physical illness may be cured by rational or scientific medicine, but if the illness or misfortune is irrational or imagined, then it may be better treated through irrational methods and the fears alleviated through magical means. "Scientific" medicine cannot deal with such a problem. Perhaps Western medical doctors also practise a little magic, more than their patients are aware. For the chronic crank who comes into the doctor's office with no physical ailment, the harmless "pink pill" and a little sympathy may be just the medicine needed. This of course brings up the problem of medical ethics and moral conscience for modern doctors, but for the traditional waganga who believe in witches, sorcery and the activity of the spirits, there is no conflict. Their role is to heal, and they combine all methods of therapy in fulfilling that role, be they herbal, communal, religious or magical.

5. The Making of Medicines

It is not within the scope of this study nor within my competence to analyze scientifically all the herbs and other substances used for healing in Dar es Salaam. Almost every tree, bush or grass found in the area is believed to have medicinal value of some sort. To list and classify all the trees, shrubs, and grasses of the area would require years of work for a trained botanist. The Botany department at the University of Dar es Salaam was able to identify only a few of the twenty-five plant specimens which my wife and I had collected from waganga for them. According to the Government Chemist, little new scientific medical knowledge and few new substances have been found in recent years through the analysis of traditional medicines. This does not mean that the search should not be continued or even intensified. The O.A.U. Scientific Council for Africa has held several symposia on the study of African medical plants and is trying to promote systematic research of African traditional medicines.[5]

The difficulty in trying to study traditional medicines and their use lies in the fact that waganga do not keep written records. They have no records either of the patients or of the diagnoses of their illnesses, nor is there any information available on the types and amounts of medicine given. Even to know the name of the plant used would be of little value unless the properties of the plant were studied by a team of botanists, chemists and pharmacists. Furthermore, its applications and results would need the scrutiny of a doctor, psychiatrist and anthropologist, together with the mganga, before any relevance to modern medical science could be determined. Up until now, with a few exceptions from West Africa, the waganga's medical knowledge has remained concealed in their minds and memories and has not been transmitted to others in written form.

The mganga in Dar es Salaam who uses *miti* (literally trees, but meaning also shrubs, grass, herbs as well as the roots, bark and leaves of trees) is to some degree an expert botanist. He knows the local names of numerous plants and trees found in the area and can determine which are poisonous and which have healing properties. Some *miti* have symbolic value, which is considered just as important in healing as their physical properties. Some *miti* are associated with certain spirits, and the mganga must know these associations. His information has been handed down to him orally by other waganga, through dreams, or he has just "picked it up *hivi hivi*, any old way," as one mganga explained. Sometimes during sleep the name of the medicine will be given to him for a particular illness or problem.

The difficulty in comparing the use of the medicines from one area of the country with another is that each ethnic group has a different language and hence a different name for the *miti*. The Zaramo sometimes use Zaramo and sometimes Swahili names for their plants and medicines. Unless the Latin scientific name is found, the local name is of little use to others. For this reason other studies made on local medicines in Tanzania were of little help. A number of anthropologists and doctors have made investigations in their regions, but their material was never followed up with additional study and a chemical analysis of the plants listed.[6] The East Africans Herbarium, located in Nairobi, Kenya, is equipped to classify plants sent to them, but at the time of this study there were not the facilities nor funds for an ongoing programme of chemical analysis.

While the waganga may be expert botanists, they know relatively little about the body and the possible physical malfunctions and diseases. The number of diseases they are able to identify are few. Fortunately they can recognize tuberculosis and leprosy and will normally recommend that the client should go to a government hospital for treatment. Waganga have no particular resentment of Western medicine and doctors and will go to a clinic or hospital for treatment if they are unable to cure themselves. They like to compare themselves to "European" doctors, saying that both groups "do medicine;" they specialize in "African" medicine and diseases and the others in "European" diseases.

In making local medicine a mganga knows that certain plants have properties that help fevers and stomach pains. But waganga have other factors which they consider just as important in the making of the medicine. For example, the color of the garment worn when cutting the *miti*, medicinal plants, the time of day and the position of the moon must also be taken into account. Some *dawa*, medicine, to be effective, must be prepared while the mganga is naked. Some *dawa* receives special power when it is placed in contact with male or female sexual organs. Some 'love medicines', or medicines used to attract customers into beer bars are said to be first placed in a woman's vagina before use. The power of the medicine for most waganga lies not in its chemical property but in the power of the waganga and their skill in preparing it properly.

Waganga seldom use only one type of *miti* for a particular medicine. Most medicines contain several different herbs and roots. If a client returns several times to the same doctor he may be given different medicine at each visit. It would be very difficult to study the results of traditional medicine because it would be difficult to know which of the many herbs were actually therapeutic. Even if a herb had medicating properties, the mganga might consider it useless unless applied with the proper ritual and prayers. The number seven is the ritual number for the Zaramo. A mganga might walk around a tree seven times before taking the root or bark and may ask the client to drink or apply the medicine seven times.

Some Zaramo believe that the mganga has within himself some inherent power which becomes operative when he makes and administers the *dawa*. Both the client and the mganga believe the cure is not dependent on the medicating properties of the *dawa* alone, but also on the power and skill of the mganga as he counteracts the supernatural forces which caused the illness. The mganga must fight this power of sorcery or the spirit or *jini* with his stronger power. If the illness cannot be overcome, the mganga will often admit to the client that the sorcerer simply had stronger medicine than he, or that his *dawa* cannot overcome *jini* or particular coastal or foreign spirits. Herbs and roots are not sufficient in themselves, but must be accompanied by the proper words and rituals and only then do they become what we call traditional medicine.

It is this mixture of herbs and magic which makes the study of traditional medicine so difficult. More often than not, the *miti* used is powerless to cure, but through psychosomatic processes, a healing eventually takes place. Or it may be an illness induced through fear of sorcery which is alleviated through magical means. Very real fears and tensions are relieved through protective medicines and amulets. The religious factor, which is neither easy to comprehend nor to appraise, must also be included. Incantations of a religious nature calling on God, on traditional spirits or on ancestors, often precede the giving of the herbal prescription. Readings from the Koran or other Muslim writings or the drinking of rose water fall into the category of a therapeutic spiritual faith healing method. The importance of the rose water or the burning of *ubani*, incense, may have some psychological effect and importance to the believer which we cannot measure. The spiritual factor does not lend itself to any systematic investigation but its importance all the same must not be underestimated.

It may be at this psychosomatic level that African medicine has kept a healing dimension which is lacking in purely "scientific" medicine. An increasing number of studies in Western medicine are discussing the importance of the body-psyche and spiritual approach to healing.[7] In a number of large hospitals; doctors, psychiatrists and pastors work as teams with better results than with only a physiological approach to the medicine. In this regard the African mganga in Dar es Salaam takes on all three roles, being the doctor, the psychiatrist and the priest, all in one. It is easy to point out the areas of magic and unscientific procedures, but the fact remains that thousands of people return to the waganga in Dar es Salaam each day because they find that their medicine seems to work.

In Dar es Salaam tree roots, leaves and herbs are generally collected from the bush and forest areas by the individual mganga or his helper. With a few exceptions he collects them himself, and when his stock runs low he returns to the bush or forest to replenish the supply. In the rural areas it is more common for the mganga to collect the medicine for the particular client and his problem, case by case. This does not work in the city because of the distances and the number of patients queuing daily in the waiting room. So the mganga keeps a supply of medicine on hand.

Roots of trees and shrubs, and bark from trees, are more commonly used than leaves or seeds. The fact that the expression *dawa ya miti*, medicine of trees, is used to cover all herbal medicines perhaps indicates that the tree is one of the main sources of medicine rather than grass, berries or seeds, although the word *miti* is used locally also to mean stems of any kind of plant.

Medicines are prepared by three basic methods: boiling, pounding and burning. Roots, bark and leaves of trees are generally boiled, although leaves can be soaked in water without boiling - the resulting "juice" then being applied externally as a kind of water treatment. Usually, several different kinds of roots are boiled together. For some treatments the vapor from these roots is inhaled while the water is boiling. The water may be drained off from the roots and leaves and drunk as medicine or used for bathing, depending on the mganga's advice. In some cases the same medicine may be inhaled, drunk and used for bathing.

The following are a few examples of this boiled type of medicine:

1. The leaves of the following trees and plants are put into a *nyungu*, clay pot: *mzizima*, *mseka*, *mvula*, *mvugula* and *mtete*. Also added are *mkunde*, runner beans. These beans are often used as a basic food substance with which medicine is boiled or later mixed. Because *uji* is red in color, it has symbolic qualities. (*Uji*, a maze meal, cooked and served as a thin gruel, is also a base food into which medicine is mixed and eaten.) The above mentioned leaves are boiled together and the medicine is called *mnuke*, Sw. vapor, steam. This medicine is first inhaled as vapor while it is boiling, and after it is cooked the leaves are separated and the water is drunk as medicine. This medicine is said to cure those troubled and ill from *shetani*, bad spirits. *Shetani* in this context does not correspond to the English words Satan or devil. Amongst the Zaramo such spirits by name are usually Kinyamkera or Mwenembango, but *shetani* could mean any inland spirit as well as *jini*, the coastal Arab spirits.

2. The root from a creeping plant with thick leaves, *sagamba*, is pounded and pulverized in a mortar, then boiled and drunk. This medicine is used to cure illness caused by the Zaramo spirit Mwenembago. The leaves of this plant are used for boils. The plant is also used in the rites connected with the Zaramo initiation camp.

3.The root from the tree *kiguti cha buga* is boiled and drunk for *chango*, stomach trouble. Any illness or disturbance in the stomach area is called chango. In most cases it is thought to be caused by sorcery. The symptoms seem to be similar to stomach ulcers, worms or various indigestion problems.[8]

4. The leaves of the *mpugupugu* are pounded into the powder form, mixed and boiled with water and then drunk.[9] This is used to cure stomach troubles. This medicine was prescribed to a mganga by her dead father in a dream after several other local medicines had failed to bring relief to her client.

5. *Madohola*, Z. (*Kudohola*, Z. to open), *mbaazi*, Sw., *Cajanus cajan*, L. pigeon pea. Roots of *madohola* are boiled in water which is then drunk as medicine. It causes diarrhoea and it is thought to remove the witchcraft substance from the body. This medicine is used when the whole body aches (from sorcery). From the leaves of this plant a medicine is made for ulcerous cracks and sores on the feet called *nyungunyungu*, S.

6. *Kinyele*, Z. medicine to stop a child crying. The roots of a plant called *kinyele*, Z. are boiled and the water is given to the baby to drink and also to be bathed in. This will stop the baby from crying. The preparation of this medicine is also important. The informant advised, "When going to dig the root you must be quiet and not talk to anyone. You have to boil it quietly, and when you bath the baby and give it to it to drink you must also be quiet."

7. Protection medicine. The following items were required by a Muslim mwalimu/mganga living in Ilala, in order to make protection medicine: $1/2$ kilo coffee beans, 40 cents worth of salt, one rooster, one tail from a fish called *pweza*, $1/4$ liter simsim seeds, seven needles, $1/2$ kilo *ulezi* grain, $1/2$ liter millet, *ubani*, incense - 40 cents worth, a small pot, 30 cents worth of peppers and one *kitunguu saumu*, garlic onion. The ingredients were to be boiled.

Medicines in powder form are also commonly used. A medicine man's bag will contain a number of small gourds containing various powders. These powders vary a great deal in content. Some are made from ashes of leaves and grass, others from pounded bones or various grains. The applications of such powders also vary. Some powdered medicines are put in boiling water and are drunk. Some are eaten orally: they are given to the client on the palm of his hand to be licked up with the tongue. Sometimes treatments will call for small incisions to be made on the forehead, arms, stomach or wherever the pain is located. Into these cuts the powdered medicines will be rubbed.

The mganga usually wishes to keep the contents of most powered medicines as his secret. He will generally tell the names of the trees and leaves he uses, but seldom the content of his powders. However one Zaramo mganga with whom my wife and I had gained particular confidence agreed to give us not only a sample of his powdered medicines but to take us to the cemetery where he claimed to dig up dead bodies with which to make certain types of medicines. So one moonlit night we accompanied Mganga M.S. on a journey into the forest, not knowing what it would lead to.

Before beginning the midnight walk the mganga brought out two small gourds, *tumba*, containing protective medicine for the journey. The first was a black gourd with a string of porcupine quills strung around the middle. From the gourd he poured out some white powder and rubbed it on his and our elbows and in the elbow pits. Over the powder he rubbed what smelled like coconut oil. The second gourd had two strings of white beads around the narrow neck and one string of green beads. Encircling the gourd at the wider base was an ivory bracelet made from elephant tusk. From this gourd he pulled out the long top stopper and dabbed the liquid medicine on the bottom of our bare feet. In addition to this "strong preventative medicine" he took a lamp, a *panga*, machete, and an old *bunduki*, gun. The gun, he explained, was his *tambiko* - his heirloom from his ancestors. His wife volunteered that he would get sick if he did not carry it. It was an old gun made by a local locksmith a few generations back and did not work any more.

After three-quarters of an hour's walk in the forest and bush country we came to a place where he left his lamp and *panga* and proceeded into a clearing where we could see by the moonlight a small Muslim graveyard with the typical slab stones at the head and foot of each grave. The mganga called out in a clear voice to the dead spirits to let them know we were coming. Then he made an oral prayer to the spirits telling them not to harm us white people because we were good ones who would do no harm to them, nor disturb them; and that they should not disturb us. We really expected the mganga to start digging a grave, as he had said he would do before the journey. Instead of that, he pulled from his pocket two small bottles of powdered medicine which he handed to us. He explained that the medicine had come from bodies in this graveyard that he had dug up on an earlier occasion.

Later in the night after we had returned to the mganga's house, he explained these two medicines and several others as follows:

1. *Mwenda kaburi*, Sw. (one who goes to a grave). Contains grey powder made from the human brain, not from the bone or hair but the brain substance itself, *ubongo*, Sw. The brain powder, he explained, is not to be ground by a human being but is found in this powder form inside the skull in the grave.

2. *Majaribu*, Sw. (trials), made from the tibia, leg shin bone of a human. The bone is pounded into a white powder. About 1/2 teaspoon is eaten dry when a person has been bewitched, *akishalogwa.*

3. *Muhambalasha*, a root which is dried and ground into powder. Two spoonfuls of powder are put into cold water. It is used *mambo ya kike, siku za mwezi, kuumwa mwezi* (for "women's problems"), at the time of menstruation, especially when bleeding does not stop but continues from month to month.

4. *Mkulwi (mkulewi)*, a pinkish powder made from the root of a tree called *mkulwi, Cassia petersiana* L.[10] The root is dried in the sun and then pounded into the powder form. This powder is boiled in the water and then strained when put into bottles. Two spoonfuls should be taken in the morning and evening for sharp stomach pains.

5. *Mpuva*, Z., *Caesalpinia crista*, L., a dark brown powder made from the root of a *mpuya* tree. The powder is boiled in the water and drunk when cooled. It is used for curing *soloka* and *mgola*, Z. (gonorrhea and syphilis). The Mwera also cook shavings from the root as a cure for gonorrhea while the Yao eat powdered leaves for severe pains in the stomach.

The above medicines in powder form are dry and have been made either from roots or dry bones. Some medicines are produced by pounding in order to extract juice. The following is an illustration of this type of medicine: *Hembebala* Z. (to blow out misfortune). The leaves of the hembebala plant are pounded in order to extract the juice. This is then taken in order to remove any substance in the body put there by witchcraft. It causes severe diarrhoea which is later rectified by drinking coconut milk. This is said to be a poisonous plant which can cause blindness, a bad rash and can even kill a person.

The medicines numbered 1-5 above were explained to me by one medicine man as a sample of what he uses. Another mganga might use the same root or leaf but call it by a different name and use it for a different purpose. Waganga of another tribe would again have different names and uses for the same root or herb. Until very much systematic and scientific investigation is made on each particular medicine by chemists, botanists, pharmacists and anthropologists as a team, little value can be drawn from these descriptions for modern medicine. Until now very little has been done along these lines except by the Government Chemists who mainly analyze cases of poisoning when brought in by the Police for autopsy. Although from time to time there is a popular public cry in Tanzania to glorify traditional medicine, its defenders would have little support from the Government Chemist, who must daily analyze the dead bodies brought in due to the medicines given by waganga. In the early 1970s there were between 400-500 poisoning cases examined each year. This only represented the small number brought into Dar es Salaam by the Police for examination. There must be a large number of people who die either from medicine given or because they do not receive medical attention and are buried without investigation.

Whether the 400-500 death cases brought in for examination represent an increase in poor traditional medicine or a better police investigation system cannot be determined. It could even represent an increase in the number of waganga practising and in clients, due to normal population growth. The Chief Government Chemist, Mr. Khomo, in a lecture at the University College, Dar es Salaam, in 1968, suggested that the knowledge of traditional "native medicine" is decreasing, waganga are forgetting good herbal remedies because they were not written down and improved upon over the years as had happened in Europe.

One ingredient recently added to the traditional medicines which, according to the Government Chemist, causes deaths or serious illness, is agricultural insecticides. Waganga reason that if insecticides can kill insects and rodents in the field they ought to be able to kill "bugs" in the body. Agricultural insecticides are cheap in price and come conveniently in powdered form, which makes them easy to add to traditional medicine, with dire results.

Altogether, 77 medicines were described to me by the waganga. The waganga who gave this information had many years of experience in the practice and discussed their medicines with professional assurance that these were time-tested, efficacious medicines.

To sum up the uses of the 77 medicines, taking into account that some of them are used for varied purposes, the following list can be made:

Spirit rites and spirit caused diseases	19	Naming rites	4
General illness and pain	15	Diarrhoea	3
Stomach pain and trouble	12	Eyes	3
Sorcery	11	Gonorrhea	2
Protection	5	Ear ache	2
Boils or sores	4	Fever	2

In addition, one medicine was given for each of the following uses: cough, abortion, menstruation, toothache, baby crying, bad dreams, contraception and love potions.

This list indicates the wide range of specific illnesses and troubles the waganga are prepared to treat. A little over one-half of the medicines are used for curing physical illnesses (49), while less than one-half (40) are medicines for non-physical illnesses, in cases concerning such matters as spirits, protection, sorcery, love potions and dreams.

The wide mixture of herbal and magical medicines and the many non-physical problems dealt with by the waganga make their function in the urban society more comprehensive than government-directed Ministry of Health programmes can offer. The mixture of herbal and magical medicines makes it difficult to built up a government-recognized system which would at least partly be based on the traditional methods of cure and therapy. If it were only a matter of improving the herbal extractions and teaching some methods of measuring the dosages given to the patients, or keeping records of diagnoses and results, there might be possibilities to upgrade the waganga and use their services until a time when the country has sufficient hospitals and trained staff. But the question involves also traditional religious beliefs, Koranic forms of healing and a non-scientific concept of illness, its cause and methods of cure. It is in these areas that it is difficult to give government sanction and make use of the medicine man's services without serious reservations.

To illustrate how a mganga may use a variety of medicines, both herbal and magical, to cure and protect his clients I shall give the following account of an observed case:

> Ndugu N.G., a Zaramo local magistrate, suddenly became ill. He went to the hospital doctor the first day and received an injection. His condition did not improve. His wife went on the morning of the second day to a traditional diviner. The mganga/diviner revealed that Ndugu N.G. had been hit by a *jini*. She was told it was the work of a woman who left a *jini* in their bathing room to attack him. It was supposed to make him mad and kill him, but it had not worked well and it only went to his head. The man's brother went to get a mganga to cure him at home as he was too weak to get up. The mganga arrived at 2:30 p.m. with a basket full of leaves, roots, small pieces of sticks and bottles.
>
> The mganga stood quietly and smelled the room for five minutes. Then he sat down on the floor mat and produced three large red *hirizi*, amulets, from his pocket. They were old and dirty. He held them on his left arm and began to whisper words to them which were inaudible to the others in the room. Then he ordered Ndugu N.G.'s wife to boil a pot of water. When the water was boiling he took brown powdered medicine from a bottle and poured it into the pot. An assortment of different kinds of leaves were taken from his basket and put into the pot and left boiling for thirty minutes. From time to

time he held his three *hirizi* and whispered words to them. He explained later that the *hirizi* revealed to him what medicines to use. Also, if there is anything bad caused by *uchawi*, sorcery, they will warn him. Even if he is walking on the road, his *hirizi* will tell him if anything bad is ahead of him.

The mganga then ordered the patient to get out of bed and sit on the floor facing east. With a spoon made from a coconut shell he dipped one large spoonful of the brewed medicine and gave it to the client's sister to give to the patient. He was to drink only part of it and the rest the sister was to rub over his body. When this was done the mganga ordered them to cover Ndugu N.G. with a white bed-sheet. The boiling pot of medicine was placed under the sheet with the patient, and he sat in the steam for ten minutes. Following this the mganga ordered more water to be boiled, into which he placed a new assortment of roots for about twenty minutes. While the medicine was cooling he ordered the family to bring pieces of red and black cloth. Into the black cloth he mixed three types of powder taken from his medicine bag. Their colors were red, brown, and black. The ends of the black cloth were tied to keep the medicine from spilling out. With the red cloth, the medicine bag was tied to Ndugu N.G.'s left arm.

When the boiled root medicine had cooled, the mganga took one cupful, into which he mixed some brown powder and gave it to the patient to drink. After this he told the client to lie on his bed, for he would soon begin to vomit, commenting, "We shall see what will come out." The mganga assured the relatives present not to worry because everything would be all right.

Within forty minutes Ndugu N.G. began to vomit violently, and continued to do so until he became unconscious. All were asked to leave the room until the vomiting stopped. While Ndugu N.G. remained unconscious, the mganga mixed green leaves from his basket with water in a pot and began to sprinkle the floor, windows, doors and everyone who was in the room. At about 8:30 p.m. the mganga asked the patient's wife to prepare food for Ndugu N.G., for he would be hungry when he woke up. The patient, however, slept through the night.

The third day the mganga was still present treating his client. He tied amulets on both arms and legs and about the patient's neck. This was to make the client dream. In the dream he would see who had bewitched him and who were his enemies. The mganga assured his client that the *jini* had now left him and he was out of danger. Had they not called him so quickly, he indicated the client would have been mad by now for it was a strong and dangerous *jini* which went to his head.

Again the mganga boiled a pot of roots and gave the medicine to Ndugu N.G. to drink. The client was better on the fourth day, and completely well on the seventh day. The mganga charged Shs. 65/- for the medicines and Shs. 100/- for the protection medicines and amulet.

This account shows the variety of medication used by the mganga. There were powdered medicines, green leaves, roots and sticks. The medicine was prepared in boiling water or in cold water. It was used for drinking, bathing, inhaling and rubbing on. Medicine was also worn about the arms, legs and neck. Amulets were made from herbs and used with secret words. At no time did the mganga use words from the Koran or other Muslim readings, unless his secret word-formula was such. The cure included medicine to induce vomiting and dreams. Except for the powdered medicines, all other medications used were prepared in the presence of the client and relatives. The manner and authority with which the mganga worked at his *uganga*, and the knowledge he appeared to have of the various leaves and roots, gave confidence to all around him. Both the sick client and the relatives were pleased with his skill in making medicines and his attentive services, as well as with the results.

6. The Methods of Cure Used by Dar es Salaam Medicine Men

Table 2 on the following pages lists the general types of cures used by the medicine men in Dar es Salaam. Following the general listing I shall give a brief analysis.

Ninety-three medical practitioners were interviewed in Dar es Salaam regarding their methods of treatment. In Chapter 4 the actual day's case load for 60 of these 93 practitioners will be analyzed. Eighty-four of the 93 were traditional medicine men, while nine were Muslim clerics, either *shehe* or *mwalimu*, who in addition to their therapeutic practise were leaders of a mosque or were Koran school teachers. Their therapeutic practise was not unlike that of the traditional waganga except that all used the Koran in treatment and all practised divining. Four, however, used both the Koran and herbal treatment.

TABLE 2: Treatment Methods Used by Medicine Men and Muslim Clerics in Dar es Salaam

Description of Practice						Methods Used in Treatment							
No.	Case No.	Sex	Tribe	Religion	General type of medicine practiced	Koran	Amulets	Herbs	Smoke treatment	Vapor treatment	Exorcism	Divines	Takes Mental Cases
A: Medicine Men													
1	K.1	M	Za	Mu	H & B	*	*		*				
2	K.2	M	Za	Mu	B	*	*		*			*	
3	K.3	M	Za	Mu	H & B	*	*	*	*			*	
4	K.5	M	Za	Mu	H		*	*	*				
5	K.7	M	Za	Mu	H			*				*	
6	K.8	M	Ny	Mu	H		*	*	*				
7	K.9	M	Za	Ch	H			*					
8	K.10	F	Za	Mu	H & S		*				*		
9	K.11	M	Za	Mu	H & B	*		*					
10	K.12	M	Za	Mu	H			*				*	*
11	K.20	M	Za	Mu	B	*						*	
12	K.21	M	Za	Mu	H & B	*		*				*	
13	K.22	M	Za	Mu	B	*	*		*	*		*	
14	K.23	M	Za	Mu	H		*	*	*	*		*	*
15	T.1	M	Ru	Mu	H & B	*	*	*	*	*			*
16	T.2	M	Ma	Mu	H & B	*	*	*	*	*		*	*
17	T.3	M	Ar	Mu	B	*	*		*			*	*
18	T.5	M	Za	Mu	Mz & H		*	*	*	*		*	*
19	M.1	M	Za	Mu	B	*	*		*	*		*	
20	Mt.1	M	Kw	P	H & S			*	*	*	*	*	
21	O.1	F	Ng	Mu	Mz & H		*	*	*	*			
22	I.0	M	Zw	Mu	H		*	*	*				
23	I.1	M	Ru	Mu	H & B	*	*	*	*			*	
24	I.2	M	Kw	Mu	H		*	*	*				
25	I.3	M	Ku	Mu	H		*	*	*				
26	I.4	M	Za	Mu	H		*	*	*				
27	I.5	M	Ru	Mu	H		*	*	*				
28	I.7	M	Sw	Mu	H			*	*				
29	1.8	M	Ru	Mu	H & B	*	*	*	*				
30	1.9	M	Za	Mu	H		*	*	*				
31	1.10	M	Za	Mu	H		*	*	*				
32	1.11	M	Ku	Mu	H		*	*	*				
33	1.12	M	Za	Mu	B	*	*		*				*
34	1.13	M	Lu	Mu	H		*	*	*				
35	1.14	M	Za	Mu	H		*	*	*				
36	1.15	M	Za	Mu	H & Mz			*	*	*		*	
37	1.17	M	Za	Mu	H		*	*	*				
38	1.18	M	Za	Mu	H			*	*				
39	1.19	M	Za	Mu	H & B	*	*	*	*				*
40	1.20	M	Za	Mu	H		*	*					*
41	1.21	M	Za	Mu	H		*	*	*				
42	1.22	M	Ru	Mu	H & B	*	*	*	*				
43	1.23	M	Za	Mu	H & B	*	*	*	*				
44	1.24	M	Ma	Mu	H		*	*	*	*			
45	1.25	M	Za	Mu	H		*	*	*				
46	1.26	M	Za	Mu	H & B	*	*	*	*				
47	1.27	M	Lu	Mu	H		*	*	*			*	
48	1.28	M	Ma	Mu	H		*	*	*			*	
49	1.29	M	Za	Mu	H			*	*				

TABLE 2: Cont.

						Description of Practice	Methods Used in Treatment						
No.	Case No.	Sex	Tribe	Religion	General type of medicine practiced	Koran	Amulets	Herbs	Smoke treatment	Vapor treatment	Exorcism	Divines	Takes Mental Cases
50	1.30	M	Za	Mu	H & S		*	*	*		*		*
51	1.31	M	Za	Mu	H		*	*	*				
52	1.32	M	Ru	Mu	H & B	*	*	*	*			*	*
53	1.33	M	Ru	Mu	B	*	*						*
54	1.34	M	Za	Mu	B	*	*	*					
55	1.36	M	Za	Mu	H		*	*					
56	1.39	M	Za	Mu	H			*	*				
57	1.40	M	Ru	Mu	B	*	*	*	*	*		*	*
58	1.41	M	Za	Mu	H		*	*	*	*			*
59	1.42	M	Za	Ch	H			*					
60	1.43	M	Za	Mu	B	*							
61	B.0	M	Ny	Mu	H		*	*	*				
62	B.1	M	Za	Mu	H		*	*	*				
63	B.2	M	Ru	Mu	H & B	*	*	*	*				
64	B.3	M	Za	Mu	H			*	*	*		*	
65	B.4	M	Kw	Mu	H & S		*	*	*		*	*	
66	B.5	M	Za	Mu	H & S		*	*	*	*	*		
67	B.6	M	Za	Mu	H & B	*		*	*				
68	B.7	M	Za	Mu	H & B	*	*	*				*	*
69	B.8	M	Kw	Mu	H & S		*	*	*		*	*	
70	B.10	M	Za	Mu	H & S		*	*	*	*	*		*
71	B.11	M	Za	Mu	H & S		*	*	*	*	*		
72	B.12	M	Ni	Mu	H		*	*	*	*		*	*
73	B.13	M	Ny	Mu	H		*	*	*	*		*	*
74	B.14	M	Za	Mu	H		*	*	*	*			
75	B.15	M	Za	Mu	H		*	*	*	*			
76	B.16	M	Sw	Mu	H & B	*	*	*	*	*		*	*
77	B.17	M	Ny	Mu	H		*	*	*	*		*	*
78	B.18	M	Za	Mu	H & B	*	*	*	*			*	*
79	B.19	M	Kw	Mu	H & S		*	*	*		*	*	*
80	O.1	M	Ng	Mu	H & S		*	*	*		*	*	*
81	O.2	M	Po	Mu	H		*	*	*			*	
82	O.3	M	Ng	Mu	H		*	*	*			*	
83	Mz.11	M	Za	Mu	Mz & S						*		
84	Mz.5	M	Za	Mu	Mz & H		*	*	*			*	
B. Muslim Clerics													
85	MK.1	M	Sw	Mu	B	*	*		*			*	*
86	MK.2	M	Ru	Mu	B & H	*	*	*	*			*	
87	MK.3	M	Za	Mu	B	*	*					*	
88	MK.4	M	Sw	Mu	B & H	*	*	*	*			*	
89	MK.5	M	Ru	Mu	B & H	*	*	*	*			*	
90	MK.6	M	Ru	Mu	B & H	*	*	*				*	
91	MK.7	M	Za	Mu	B	*	*					*	
92	MK.8	M	Za	Mu	B	*	*					*	
93	MK.9	M	Za	Mu	B & Mz	*	*					*	

EXPLANATION OF SYMBOLS IN THE TABLE

Sex: M - male; F - female

Tribe: Za - Zaramo; Ru - Rufiji; Kw - Kwere; Ni - Ngoni; Sw - Swahili; Ny - Nyamwezi; Ma - Makua; Ng - Ngindo; Ku - Kutu; Lu - Luguru; Po - Pogoro; Ar - Arab

Religion: Mu - Muslim; Ch - Christian; P - Kipazi (Zaramo traditional religion)

Type of Medicine Practised: H - *Dawa ya miti*, Herbal; B - *Dawa ya Kitabu*, Medicine of the book, Koran and other Islamic writings; S - Spirit exorcism (*madogoli, rungu* etc.); Mz - *Mzimu*, spirit shrines, graves or huts.

There are four basic forms of treatment and each of these is normally administered to the client by several different methods. The majority, that is 77 of the 93 practitioners, use herbs. Thirty-seven use the Islamic books, eleven can cure by exorcising spirits, while six treat their clients through prayer and the ritual offerings at the spirit hut, usually located beneath a large baobab tree. Prayers and ritual at the *mzimu* hut are never used alone but always together with one of the other forms of treatment. Of the six *mzimu* hut keepers, four also gave herbal treatments and one used the *mzimu* and the Koran.

Of the 77 practitioners who used herbs, 41 or over half used only herbs, while 22 used herbs and the book, 19 used herbs and exorcism rites (*madogoli*), and 4 used herbs and *mzimu* spirit shrines. Of the 37 who used Koran for treatment, 14 used the Koran alone, while 22, as stated above, used the Koran and herbs, and one used the Koran and a *mzimu* spirit shrine.

When herbs and the Koran are used, they may be administered to the client by several different methods, as has been shown. Boiling the herbs, after which the water is drunk by the client, is the most common method and was said to be practised by all 77 herbal users.

Seventy-three waganga said they gave smoke treatments. Herbs or pieces of paper with verses of the Koran written on them are burnt over a charcoal fire, the smoke of which is inhaled by the client. Twenty-two practitioners said they administer the vapor treatment, which consists of putting herbs into boiling water after which the client sits with the pot under a cloth and inhales the vapor.

Eleven of the 93 waganga were able to treat their clients by performing the *madogoli* exorcism rites. Although 11 of the waganga were able to give such treatment, it is usually performed in the countryside and not in the city. Only occasionally is it done in Buguruni. The urban waganga may take their clients to a country area for the *madogoli*, but more often they leave this type of treatment for the rural waganga to perform. As will be seen in the study of the waganga's case loads, spirit possession is one of the urban Zaramo's lesser ailments, while it is the most frequent problem for their country kin.

Twenty-four of the waganga took on mental cases, whose treatment might consist of a combination of herbal, Koranic, vapor and smoke methods, as well as the wearing of amulets. Amulets were made and administered by 77 waganga, the same number as administered herbal treatments. Inside the amulet may be placed either powdered herbs or a piece of paper with Koranic verse written on it. Pieces of various bones, seeds or wood may also be enclosed in an amulet. None of the medicine men said they limit their practice to the making of amulets. It was always combined with other methods of treatment.

It may be noted in Table 2, that 41 of the 93 practitioners diagnosed their clients' problems through the art of divination (see Chapter 3). In relation to the types of treatment given, it may be said here that more diviners were found amongst those who gave treatment by herbal methods than amongst those who used the Islamic book method.

There has been a gradual penetration of Islamic elements into the older Zaramo traditional practices. At the same time , the traditional beliefs have modified Islamic practices, so that often no clear borderline can be drawn between these different origins. The fact that the mganga in his practice combines both elements makes him acceptable to a wider circle of clients than would be the case if he stuck to only one way. It also indicates a need for a balance of power control of forces of different kinds. This reflects the growing cultural and religious integration taking place in the coastal and urban Zaramo society.

Raymond Prince states that the Yoruba of Nigeria have three explanations for the cause of illness and misfortune, i.e. the natural, the preternatural and the supernatural (1964, 88). He says that for the natural physical cause the medicine man will give a herbal treatment. For preternatural causes such as curse, witchcraft and sorcery, he will carry out a magical act to counter the evil power. For supernatural causes, such as the various types of spirits, he may ask the client to make a ritual sacrifice or offering or to go through an exorcism. These three casual categories are believed in by Zaramo also, and we shall see in the waganga case material that they use identical methods to handle such cases. For the natural causes, 77 out of 93 medicine men used herbs. For the preternatural causes, smoke and vapor treatments, amulets and the Koran were used by the majority of the waganga. For the supernatural, exorcism and *tambiko* [11] ritual offerings were used. One or all of these methods may be needed to complete the cure and therefore we see in the evidence that most medicine men use two or more methods of treatment. By combining the various types of treatment the mganga recognizes the physical, social and supernatural causes of illness and misfortune.

7. Payments Involved in Traditional Healing Services

One of the most sensitive areas of enquiry in this study was the question of payments for *dawa* and *uganga* services. The clients displayed no reluctance about disclosing how much they paid in fees for treatment by waganga, but the waganga themselves were frequently averse to discussing this. Most questions they answered freely, but when touching upon payment of fees several either refused to answer or commented ambiguously that "people give what they like or what they are able."

Within this study 29 waganga were willing to tell what they charge for various medicines and services, and 27 clients listed payments they had made for a variety of treatments. These two groups of figures tend to correspond fairly well, except that the waganga preferred to state an indefinite amount such as between 10 and 20 shillings or between 100 and 200 shillings rather than a fixed price. It is very likely that waganga were being truthful, as payments often vary according to the clients' financial means.

The waganga apparently appraise their clients' economic status by the manner in which they dress and conduct themselves. It can be assumed that a well-dressed office worker, for example, would be charged a higher rate than a barefoot peasant. At the beginning of my research I noticed that the clients listed higher fees when the enquiry was made by me personally, while lower rates were recorded by my assistants. Therefore I refrained from dealing with financial questions myself.

Throughout the interviewing period I found no one who complained about the high price of traditional medicine. It seemed that people expect to pay a good price for "powerful medicine." If it costs nothing they consider it to be worthless. Furthermore, I found no evidence in Dar es Salaam of the system whereby treatment is given without prepayment, the client only coming back to pay if and when he is cured as has been reported to be the practice in other ethnic groups. A number of respondents said, however, that they paid 20 or 30 shillings and if the treatment was particularly effective they returned to give an extra thank-offering. Even in the cases of unemployed persons seeking work, between 20 and 35 shillings was charged, not an insignificant sum for a person with no income.

Only when the medicine failed completely to bring the expected results did some persons complain of being cheated. But this did not discourage them from consulting other waganga. The general impression was that people were satisfied with the services and medicine of the waganga and therefore were willing to pay fairly substantial sums of money rather than attend a government hospital. It was often said in the past that people preferred to go to Christian "mission" hospitals because they were charged a small fee, whereas the government hospitals charged nothing. The implication was that the government medicine was not as good because it was free of charge. Similarly it may be that people have more confidence in traditional medicine because it is so costly.

The lowest charge listed was for divining, which ranged from two to four shillings. The most expensive treatment was that for mental illness, with protection and treatment for sorcery following behind. Mentally ill patients attended several sessions over a period of weeks and the price given covered the full treatment, not per session treatment. Prison and court cases were also costly, but there were very few brought to the waganga for treatment. The extraordinary element here is that seemingly poverty-stricken people can find the money to pay such rates.

The staggering conclusion one must draw from this information is that most waganga practising in Dar es Salaam are exceptionally wealthy men. Well established waganga can afford to own several houses and support several wives. For example, the average number of cases treated by the traditional mganga per day is twelve. If as the payment survey revealed 42/60 shillings is the average payment received per client, the mganga's daily income is 511/20 shillings, a wage almost unheard of for Tanzania. Even if his income were only half that amount it would equal that of a Tanzanian Government minister's salary. Or, if he received only 10 shillings per client, the very lowest total fee actually paid, he would be still averaging 120/- shillings per day, equal to that of a university professor. It is possible to understand then why one mganga in Ilala could own eleven houses and why another could afford a large car with a chauffeur.

While government medical funds are limited and hospital staff are grossly overworked, the traditional mganga enjoys a light case load of twelve patients per day on average and an income equal to, if not several times larger than that of a government doctor. Furthermore, his income is tax-free. It is almost surprising that more Tanzanians do not join this profession just for the sheer prospect of wealth.

NOTES TO CHAPTER 1

[1]Tanganyika Government, *The Laws of Tanganyika*, Vol. II, (London, Watmough Ltd., 1947), Cap. 92.20. Also found in *Tanzania Laws*, Chapter 409, Section 37; and Chapter 416, Section 53.

[2]According to the 1967 Census there were 19,122 Zaramo households in Dar es Salaam. There was an average of 3.3 persons per household, which gives a total of 63,102 Zaramo. If 35,000 of these were over 17 years of age, then at the ratio of 3:150 it would mean approximately 700 Zaramo are practising medicine men.

[3]*Madogoli* - see Glossary. The exorcism rite consists of prayers, drumming, singing, a trance state, and other activities. For a full description of the *madogoli* ritual see Swantz, M-L, 1970, 189-192, 252, 263-64, 328-29.

[4]I returned to this house in Kigogo in March 1972, in order to take a picture of it, and discovered both signs removed and the house empty.

[5]O.A.U. Scientific Council for Africa, Duplicated document L (65) 25 OAU/STRC, Lagos: 1965; Duplicated document L (67) 12, OAU/STRC, Dakar: 1968.

[6]See Bibliography: Imperato, 1966; Korischoner, 1936; Krauss, 1918; Redmayne, 1969; Tanner, 1951; Weck, 1908.

[7]See e.g. Siirala, Aarne: *The Voice of Illness*, Philadelphia; Fortress Press, 1964; Siirala, Martti: "Our changing conception of illness", *Journal of Religion and Health*, Vol. 5, No. 2, 1966, 105-118.

[8]Medicines 1-3 as told by Mganga A.O.

[9]*Mpugupugu* tree species: *Bignoniaceae* L., *Markhamia acuminata* L., and *Markhamia obtusifolia* L. These small bush-like trees grow in the thickets and dense bush, have paired leaves and long ribbon-like seedpods. They grow also in the Southern Province and are known in Nyasa, Ngindo and Matumbi languages by the same name, *mpugupugu*. Its wood is used for making handles of cultivating implements and by the Ngoni and Ngindo for making arrows. The leaves have been used for wrapping food and strips of bark for making soles for rough sandals; see Davy, J.B., 1940.

[10]Known as *mtewelewe* in Yao and *Mlewilewi* in Mwera. The tree is common throughout the Southern Province and distinguished by its long round seed pods. The fruits are edible and the Yao also use the roots to make medicines for stomach pains.

[11]In most Zaramo clans, kin groups assemble at the ancestral graves or spirit huts to make a yearly *tambiko*, ritual offering. This must not be understood to be ancestor worship or worship of spirits. At best it is to show respect to the dead through symbolic offerings and ritual which may include prayers, sacrifice, incense, and offerings of rice, *pombe* -beer, bananas and eggs. Several elders generally give the prayers, along with the family medicine men present. All kin related to the deceased should be present, or at least represented, at the yearly *tambiko*.

CHAPTER 2
Other Types of Medicine Men and Women

1. The Itinerant Waganga, Witchcraft Eradicators

Throughout East Africa, but especially in the coastal area, there are a number of itinerant waganga whose main claim to fame lies in their witch finding or witch eradicating activity.[1] When these witch finders come into Dar es Salaam and to the surrounding villages, their presence creates much excitement in the community. Many hundreds of people come to be treated or watch the excitement connected with the event.

One of the most famous itinerant witch eradicators to move about in Tanzania was the man, now deceased, called Nguvumali (Lienhardt, 1968). Although Nguvumali is dead, another medicine man has taken his name and operates today in the coastal area. This man, whose real name is Hemedi Saidi Matoroka, worked between December 1967 and January 1968 in the Dar es Salaam area. Ali, the son of the true Nguvumali now deceased, continues his father's work as an itinerant medicine man and also uses "Nguvumali" as his trade name. I have not heard that Ali is operating in Dar es Salaam, although he does come from time to time to collect the money left at his father's grave.

The following information was gathered during a week of observing the work of Matoroka, alias "Nguvumali", in several places in the city. A number of his clients were interviewed also.

Hemedi Saidi Matoroka and all his helpers are Ngindo by tribe. He himself comes from Nachingwea and his clan is Nyiponera. Matoroka said he was instructed in uganga, medicine, by Nguvumali. Part of this name, Hemedi Saidi Matoroka, is derived from the name of the deceased mganga who trained the original Nguvumali. I do not know if there is any family relationship. It is likely that he uses these names, including that of Nguvumali, in order to benefit from the reputation of these two well-known waganga. It is quite common for a novice to take for himself the name of his teacher as his "spiritual father."

Matoroka also said that he received his *uganga* through "*jadi ya mzimu* ." His is a *kumbunga* spirit, which is not a coastal spirit but rather that of an inland tribe. He has the *ngoma*, dance, of *manyanga*, referring to gourds which are round like pumpkins and which, when dried, can have inserted stones to make a rattle. Matoroka uses such a rattle in his *ramli*, divining, in order to raise the spirit to his head while singing Ngindo songs. While divining in this manner he goes into trance and an assistant interprets the spirit's voice which speaks through Matoroka. The *manyanga* rattle can also put the client into a trance and when the spirit rises the client begins to shake. Matoroka added that "the person thus treated must be a man or woman or a person who has reached the puberty stage."

Matoroka claimed that when he divines for a client he can determine whether the illness or misfortune was caused by a *jini*, by a particular spirit, or if it is the result of sorcery. He emphasized that it is inadvisable to identify or name witches, as this would cause quarrels between people. Instead, medicine is given to cure the effects of witchcraft and to protect against it. Sometimes his diagnosis is that an illness, such as tuberculosis, sores or eye troubles, should be treated in a hospital. Matoroka accepts mental patients and, "if God grants," he can cure them. For mental cases he uses only herbs which are pounded and boiled. These are drunk with water or are used when bathing.

The work for which Matoroka is most widely known is that of witchcraft eradication. Present-day laws forbid witch ordeals, in which previously a suspected person was made to drink various medicines or poisons or was asked to put his hand into boiling water to prove or disprove his being a witch. Today the strategy of Matoroka is not to detect the witch or to accuse anyone, but rather to protect his clients from the work of witches or sorcerers. Matoroka explained: *"anakula dawa sababu ya kinga"*, Sw. (He is eating medicine for the sake of protection). In other words Matoroka does not intend to be a witch finder, for which he might be taken to court by the accused, but rather to eradicate the witches and the work of sorcery by giving protective medicine.

Taking or eating anti-witchcraft medicine has several functions. First, the person taking it feels that he or she is protected. They can depart in peace, knowing that if anyone should attack them, they would be unharmed and the attacker himself would suffer. Second, to eat anti-witchcraft medicine is a testimony to the community that they themselves are not witches, nor do they practise sorcery. If people take this medicine before throwing away their witchcraft and sorcery materials it is thought that they immediately fall sick or die. The informant who told me about Mganga Songo's visit to Dar es Salaam related that she saw men drop dead after receiving the medicine and "they were carried home to be buried." Therefore, if a person is willing to eat the medicine and nothing happens, it assures the community that this neighbor is harmless. Also, if those taking the medicine should decide later to practise sorcery, the evil would return to them. This is an added comfort to the community.

Some people indicated their approval of witch eradicators who move into a community because they bring safety and peace. Sometimes innocent people, usually elderly women, are accused of practising sorcery but have no way of defending themselves or of restoring their reputation. This then is the opportunity for them to show publicly that they can eat the medicine with good conscience, proving that they have been falsely accused. The only other opportunity for a Zaramo to prove herself or himself not a sorcerer would be to make a long journey to the Uluguru Mountains to visit the *Mzimu* - Spirit Kolelo, which tests such accusation cases. Such a journey takes time and money, whereas, for a small fee and public witness by those who may suspect the person, the medicine on the tongue clears the suspicion.

The following conversation took place between two middle-aged women who appeared before Matoroka to take the anti-witchcraft medicine. The first woman said very seriously, "You say I am a *mchawi*, you see me now eat it (the medicine)." The second woman laughed and the first woman continued, "Don't laugh, I feel bitter pain because of it." She took the *dawa*, medicine, with great seriousness and then asked Matoroka if it was permissible to make medicine for planting seeds, *dawa ya kupanda*. He replied that it was all right, "for this medicine was only against *uchawi*, witchcraft."

For Christians the coming of such anti-witchcraft medicine men creates a problem. Normally they would not wish to go to such waganga, but if they do not, their neighbors accuse them of practising sorcery because they are afraid to take the medicine. For this reason many, but not all, Christians take the *dawa*.

The activity of mganga Matoroka is that of a professional who knows his business and perfected his approach to the community. Matoroka is in charge of an active team of sixteen practitioners and apprentices, four of whom are his wifes. Matoroka arrives in a village or town location riding in a large red Morris car driven by a chauffeur. Immediately upon arrival he makes arrangements with the head of the community in order to operate his business. Then he stations a team of two or three medicine men to work in that community while he establishes another group in a different section of the city or in another village. On October 27, 1967 Matoroka had a team of three working in Bunju, three in Kunduchi, his four wives and two other assistants in Kawe, and one in Kigogo. Later, when work in Bunju had finished, he moved a group into Manzese and later to Ubungo. It appears that he works the outer fringe housing areas of Dar es Salaam and not the city center areas.

Matoroka enters a community with great flair. He dresses in a red *kanzu*, robe, wearing a red turban and carrying a *msinga*, whisk, made of wildebeest tail. His assistants beat drums, sing and dance the *manyanga* to attract people. Later they line up the clients in rows in order to administer the medicine. Prior to the arrival of his assistant waganga, Matoroka makes public his coming by contacting a community TANU chairman.

When interviewed in 1967, Mganga Matoroka made every attempt to give the appearance that he not only has government approval to operate but that he is actually sent by the government to do this good work. He carried with him a framed certificate from the Division Executive Officer of Lindi, dated 1966.

At Manzese the local TANU chairman announced to the people that they should all come to receive the medicine. At Bunju, on another occasion, the TANU Divisional Officer of the area circulated a letter in the community announcing that people should make themselves available. In fact he announced a public TANU community meeting at the same time and stressed that they should come for both the meeting and the medicine. Many people are under the impression that it is a government order that they should present themselves for this medical treatment.

While at Manzese, Matoroka visited the TANU chairman's office for a twenty minute private conversation. Afterwards he made it known publicly that he was going to the Kisarawe *Boma*, district office, to get a permit, saying:"The people of Kisarawe want me, they have sent for me, so I am going to Kisarawe to get the permit." When he left, some of his helpers stayed behind and immediately began their work of drumming, singing and administering the anti-witchcraft medicine. The TANU headman led the procession, and within minutes 32 women, and 15 men and a few children had eaten the medicine. It is not known whether Matoroka actually went to Kisarawe for the permit.

After publicly administering the medicine, the waganga and apprentices withdrew to a room in the local TANU leader's house. Here people came privately for divining and to receive medicine, amulets for protection, and other forms of treatment. If a problem was too great for the assistant medicine men to solve, advice and help were received from Matoroka when he came around on one of his periodic supervisory visits. It seemed evident that money was given to the local TANU and government secretaries for their co-operation and the use of their rooms. When the business at Manzese seemed to be getting slack, the TANU chairman spoke to the curious but reluctant spectators, urging them to come for protection medicine: "This *dawa* is good for you - it is *kinga*, protection."

The social pressure upon the people to eat the medicine is very great. Those who refuse or who go away from the area until the medicine man leaves will undoubtedly be suspected of practising sorcery. But for the majority fears are relieved, as the two previous informants stated.

The charge for the Nguvumali protection medicine is minimal, only sixty cents for adults and ten cents for children.[2] Even at this low price there is substantial profit for the waganga because of the large numbers requesting the medicine. As the people assemble for treatment they are lined up in groups of ten or more. Thus arranged, they are instructed to stick out their tongues while the mganga goes down the line dabbing a little white powder from a round box on their tongues. The powder is called *usembe* and is perhaps a mixture of flour and sugar. One man indicated that it is sweet. No mganga would disclose the extract ingredients.

In observing these waganga at work on several occasions, I estimate that they were treating approximately 40 clients per working hour. In a three-hour period 60 adult men, 11 adult women, 21 youths and 29 children took the medicine. In Manzese, within one hour 15 men, 32 women and a number of small children took medicine. Some youths noticeably ridiculed the proceedings as they watched from the sidelines, but for the majority of adults between 30-50 years of age it was a serious business. When administering the witchcraft eradicating medicine, the waganga earn about 30 shillings per hour. It might be recalled that the Matoroka has three or four teams working simultaneously at this medicine, compounding his profit. In the late afternoon and evening, after the mass administration of medicine is over, clients come for *ramli*, divining, and the traditional medical treatment. Matoroka confided that between ten and twenty people come to him in an evening, and other medicine men in his team treat a similar number of clients. If each client were to pay a minimum of 10 shillings and a maximum of 50 shillings for his treatment, one medicine man could easily amass from 300 to 400 shillings per evening.

The cases reported by Matoroka and his assistants in the evening hours were not unlike those treated by other medicine men throughout the city. Six of his clients were willing to give information, but this sample is too small for an accurate assessment of his clientele and their problems. It was found that two clients were male, four were female and all were Muslims. By tribal affiliation four were Zaramo, one Zigua and one Ndengereko. Matoroka himself had divined all six cases: four cases of sickness were accredited to sorcery; one was considered a simple stomach ailment; and the sixth case was a couple who wanted children. Five clients were given medicine for a cure and in the remaining case, the couple were given protection medicine.

2. Mzimu - Spirit Shrine Keepers

Another group which I am including here are not waganga in the traditional sense, although they are often called waganga. These are the caretakers of special graves where *mzimu*, spirits, are located. These shrines or locations are visited from time to time by people seeking cures or favours of a particular kind. These graves may be of well-known medicine men, village headmen or, on the coast, ancient Shirazi or Arab notables. The caretakers lead people to the *mzimu* and sometimes offer prayers on their behalf. They also sweep the grave and collect the money left by the clients. Since the *mzimu* are a means of healing and meeting problems such as might be brought to the traditional medicine men, the *mzimu* keepers are included here as one type of medical practitioner. In some cases the shrine keepers do conduct a traditional medical practice in addition to caring for the shrine. Often, however, the title mganga is purely honorary. It should also be mentioned that many graves and trees which are visited as shrines do not have caretakers.

In Dar es Salaam I found the Zaramo going to spirit shrines at Kurasini, Mtoni, Kigogo, and Msasani, as well as to some *mzimu* outside the city area. Some examples are given here in detail.

At the time of this research, Mwalimu Yaka was the keeper of a spirit shrine called *Mwakawe* or *Mwinyikawe*, *mnyikawe*. Yaka was both the *Mwalimu*, teacher, and leader of the small mud and wattle Muslim mosque which stood near his home. His other duty was that of keeper of the *mzimu* tree of Mwakawe. Yaka, a Zaramo about 70 years of age, was both willing to talk about the *mzimu* and to show it to my wife and me.

The following account of the Kawe *mzimu* is given in the words of Mwalimu Yaka himself whom I visited several times. He died in 1970.

> Mwinyikawe was a Shirazi whose house stood where the baobab tree now stands. At that time there was a big village which surrounded the tree area. Mwakawe was a very devout Muslim who lived a long time before the "enzi ya Wadebli," the rule of the Debuls and the Wareno, the Portuguese. Mwakawe knew that these Wazungu[3], Wadeblo, *makafiri*, infidels, were coming to rule. He did not want to live under such people. He therefore prayed to God that He would not allow this to happen. "Let me sink, I and my village, because I do not want to see the *makafiri* and live under them." God heeded his prayer because he prayed this almost as a curse. God made him and his village sink into the ground. A sweet water pond was formed where Mwakawe's village stood and the baobab tree grew at the place of his house. Later people could walk by and see below the water, the people, their chickens and all their life as it continued there. Only a part of the mosque called *kibla* and a well were left on top of the ground.

The *mzimu* of Mwakawe is a large baobab tree surrounded by thick forest and underbrush. One large branch was broken and was lying near to the ground so as to form a hollow cave in the side of the trunk. A short protruding branch stump near the trunk was wrapped with cloth as a *kilemba* (turban) and from it were hanging strips of black, white and red cloth. These colors are basic Zaramo symbols, and such strips of three colors are often tied around Zaramo medicine gourds and are connected with many Zaramo rituals (Swantz, M-L., 1970, 241-255).

Mwalimu Yaka went on to tell about the use of this *mzimu* of which he was the caretaker:

People come here if they want to have work, are ill, do not have a husband or a wife, do not get children or are in need of healing or success. They come to pray and leave one shilling and give a promise to give more after the prayer has been granted, such as 30-40 shillings, a goat or other offerings. They come with a *Mwalimu* or come alone. If such a person is ill, he then goes to a mganga. When he gets what he has asked he brings what he has promised, be it *ubani*, incense, or pieces of cloth in three colors, rice, etc.

After people get what they have requested some may forget all about their promise to return to bring an offering. They then get trouble. They go for *ramli*, divining, and the *ramli* says it is because of the promise they made and did not fulfill. Then the person returns to the *mzimu* to give the promised offering, at the same time praying for the present trouble.

Some people may come and take some soil from the place for *kipandio*, to induce growth of a crop, before planting rice. Also some come for *mtego*, a trap, to put on the *shamba* so that if anyone comes to steal or harms the crops he will get very ill.

Because the man was a devout man that Mwakawe whose *dua*, prayers, were heard by God, this place has much *nguvu*, *baraka*, power and blessing. It is very powerful. Big people also come, in cars, for job protection. Some even come from Tabora, Mombasa and Tanga. They make their promise in their homes and then come when they have got what they wanted.

Mwalimu Yaka added: "The place will not be cut down. Even when the city extends this place will remain." One European had cut part of the woods to park his car and he died before the month was over.

One informant had gone to Mnyikawe *mzimu* ten years previously to request a cure for an illness. She got well but never returned. Now, after ten years when she was ailing again, she finally remembered the given promise and had come to give her offerings. Another elderly woman had gone to her ordinary family mganga with a complaint about aching legs. As nothing seemed to help she came to Mnyikawe, mentioning that the problem was *mzimu wetu*, our *mzimu*. Other members of the same family had earlier been to Mnyikawe and even she had been once before. But by calling the shrine "our" *mzimu* she also indicated that it is an Islamic shrine and not a traditional one; that it belonged to "us Muslims." Anyone can go there, but the power is conceived to be within the Islamic religious framework.

In addition to the *mzimu* tree of Mwakawe, I observed a group of baobab trees on the cliff of Kurasini creek near the oil storage installation. On this site *ubani* is burned and rituals performed. Two Zaramo men and a sick child were observed at prayer under a baobab tree near Mbagala. They were not only praying for the sick child, but also asking why he was sick.

The most famous *mzimu* grave in the Dar es Salaam area is that of Mganga Nguvumali, located in Kigogo-Minyononi area. As was mentioned earlier, Nguvumali was a well-known itinerant mganga, especially noted as a witch finder and for his potent anti-witchcraft medicine.

The main informant regarding Nguvumali was his sister. Binti M.K. was a mganga herself and attendant of Nguvumali's grave in Kigogo. Binti M.K. had learned her uganga from her brother Nguvumali, but said that he himself had travelled to many places during his youth and learned his uganga from various sources. When he returned home from his travels, he began to treat people and to catch *wachawi*, witches or wizards. Very soon he began to travel for the same purpose. Lienhardt tells that Nguvumali was an initiate of the Uliro spirit cult, which is said originally to have come from Mozambique and is considered to be an inland spirit, not one from the coast.

Binti M.K. said that she treats from ten to fifteen people each day and that she can treat any kind of trouble, including mental illness. She is known to be wealthy and owns a *duka*, a store, and a large tract of land in Kigogo which she was selling for house plots at 50 shillings each.

Binti M.K. treats her patients with traditional medicine, but people also visit the *mzimu* grave of Nguvumali with their problems. She said people go there with such problems as bad fortune, illness, loss of job, need of work, lack of children, etc. Each one who goes, leaves money on the wall of the grave. Some leave cloth or clothes hanging on the walls. No one takes the money except Ali, the son of Nguvumali, who is also an itinerant mganga and carries on his father's work.

People of all ethnic groups visit the grave, but especially the Zaramo. Binti M.K. is not willing to take people to the grave just to look at it. As she says, "I never play with my brother's grave. . . not just to take people there just like to see a picture. They must have troubles, real troubles."

Mzee K.M. is the keeper of a *mzimu*, spirit hut, built under a baobab tree in Kigogo. Mzee K.M. is a Zaramo, born at Msanga, five miles beyond Maneromango. When he moved to Kigogo in Dar es Salaam, he brought along his clan spirit, that of a young girl, and built a new hut under a baobab tree. His *mzimu*, called a "*shetani*" by the informant, belongs to the clan of Mzee K.M. Each year the clan members return to the hut to clean the area and make their yearly *tambiko*, ritual offering. Having performed these duties, the clan members sit near the hut and eat a meal of chicken and rice. They repeat the *tambiko* and meal-eating whenever they need to rebuild the hut. Clan members go to the hut for a private *tambiko* at any time of illness or special need. In such cases they must be accompanied by the owner, Mzee K.M., and must bring such things as money (5 or 10 cents), pieces of sugar cane, eggs, rice and fried millet for the offering when making the *tambiko*. Only Mzee K.M. is able to see the spirit of the young girl. He receives all the cash offerings left at the *mzimu*.

Another *mzimu* shrine is located in the Tandika area of Temeke under a large baobab tree and tended by a local mganga of that area. The following information was provided by Bibi M.R., who visits this spirit shrine.

Bibi M.R. said she was bewitched by a woman who lives in the same house. She herself does not know why this neighbor hates her. When her menstrual period did not stop after many days she went first to the clinic for medicine, but was not helped. Advised by a friend to consult a local mganga in Tandika, she went first for the *ramli*, divining, and then for the cure. According to the divining performed by the mganga, she had been bewitched by her neighbor who put *uchawi dawa*, sorcery medicine, on her door-step. She paid two shillings for the divination session. The same mganga continued with the cure.

The mganga escorted Bibi M.R. and several other clients from his house to a nearby large baobab tree. At the foot of the tree was a large shed made of *makuti*, woven palm leaves. When they reached the door the mganga spoke: "I have come my fathers; I have brought these sick people. Please God, help me, and you Mzimu, help me please. I also ask if we may come in? " There came a noise from the shed sounding like "Mmm. .mmm. .mmm."

The mganga entered first, followed by Bibi M.R. and other clients. Inside were stones arranged as a grave around which they were instructed to sit down. The mganga proceeded to make small cuts on the forehead of each client and on the back of their necks. After rubbing powder into the cuts he led the clients back to his house.

Bibi M.R. was then given *uji*, a corn meal gruel, into which the mganga had mixed medicine. After eating this she was taken from the house into a lonely area in the bush where she was left alone. After a short time she began to vomit, continuing for almost six hours until she was unconscious. About 11 p.m. she was brought back to the mganga's house, where she was given water to drink mixed with medicine. She was also given water for bathing. After this treatment she felt relatively strong again, and although she was given more medicine in a bottle to use at home, she did not drink it because she felt she was now cured. She paid 10 shillings for this medicine and treatment.

Bibi M.R. was thoroughly convinced of the power of this mganga and his *mzimu*. She said many people go there for different troubles, some waiting up to six hours to get in. She claimed to have seen even Indians and Arabs waiting to see this mganga. Bibi M.R. believed that problems of *uchawi*, sorcery, will not diminish in Dar es Salaam because those who commit sorcery have inherited the power and inclination from their fathers and grandfathers. In the conclusion she stated that she did not do any *uchawi* as revenge to the neighbor who had bewitched her.

3. Herb Sellers

In almost every society it is common knowledge that certain plants, roots and leaves have therapeutic value. This medical plant knowledge is the basis for the Zaramo traditional art of healing and constitutes the most common form of curing illness in the Zaramo society. The herbs may be given by a full-time medicine man; bought in a shop or on the street; or gathered by the patient or his/her relatives.

150 Zaramo informants were asked: *"Umetumia dawa za kienyeji ? Katika shida gani ?"* (Do you use local medicines? For what kind of troubles?). *Dawa za kienyeji* generally implies the use of herbs, but not always. It may also refer to the use of amulets, *tambiko* offerings and other traditional methods of cure which might not include herbs. Approximately 75 percent of the Zaramo do use herbs from time to time for curing bodily ills, and it is common knowledge that most adults are conversant with a number of good herbs for various ailments. They can collect and prepare the herbs for use without the aid of a medicine man. Judging from the very few places where herbs can be purchased in Dar es Salaam, it can be assumed that most Zaramo go themselves to the country to collect the herbs, plants and leaves that they wish to use.

In most open market places in cities and towns of West Africa and Southern Africa, herb sellers are found next to the vegetable and fruit stalls. In a municipal market in Salisbury I counted twelve stalls at which herbs were being sold together with a wide assortment of animal claws, skins and feathers. Individuals could purchase herbs for their private use, but the stalls were patronized primarily by local medicine men restocking their supplies. This is not the case in Dar es Salaam, where I found no herbalist stalls in the municipal market places. The waganga interviewed in Dar es Salaam all said they themselves went into the country periodically to collect supplies of roots and herbs. A few said they send an assistant or apprentice to the countryside to collect the *dawa za miti*.

There were, however, a few places in Dar es Salaam where herbs could be purchased. Near the Kariakoo market on Nyamwezi Street were two shops which specialized in herbs. Both were owned by Arabs, one having two young Tanzanian boys as attendants. The boys seemed to know very little about the use of the herbs, quoting only the price.

The Arab owner of the second shop volunteered that the herbs came from up-country as well as from Zanzibar and Mafia. Medicines from Zanzibar are always thought to be powerful. Prices ranged from one shilling to ten shillings. The Arab herb dealer had been in business at that location for twelve years. He did not divine or cure people with the herbs himself, but only sold medicine. In no sense would he be called a mganga, but rather a shopkeeper or herb seller. Also, at the corner of Uhuru and Sikukuu Streets was a shop called "Toti Store", where an Indian sold herbs.

Other herbalist street sellers were located near the Kariakoo market and at the corner of Msimbazi and Uhuru Streets. Two sellers were women of the Wakwavi tribe who sat on the side walk with a few piles of various roots displayed for sale. An old man sat on the sidewalk at the corner of Msimbazi and Uhuru Streets with another small display of roots for sale. He had been in business at the same location for eight years, indicating that this livelihood was at least adequate. Another woman sat with herbs at the corner of Msimbazi and Mhonda Streets. Again, these street sellers are not considered to be medical practitioners, but simply sellers of herbs to private users.

In view of the scarcity of stores and individuals selling herbs in Dar es Salaam, it does not appear that people often buy herbs for their own use as one would buy medicine at a chemist shop. The large number of waganga in the city indicates rather that herbs, if used, are prescribed and given to clients by these practitioners.

4. Street Sellers/Hawkers

More numerous than the herbalist street sellers or stores in Dar es Salaam are the men who sell prepared medicines in bottles on the streets of the city. In 1967 there were about 12 medicine street hawkers in Dar es Salaam organized by a central office-cum-store on Mikumi Street in Magomeni. This association was called African Native Medicines and had its "head factory" in Sindeni, Tanga District. It was run by three local medicine men: Omari A. Chepe, Iddi A. Bogu and Abdallah Mgwambi. From Sindeni the medicine was sent in large bottles to Dodoma, Iringa, Moshi, Morogoro, Ifakara, Kisarawe and Dar es Salaam. At these local points the medicine was put into small injection bottles which had been used and discarded by local government hospitals and presumably collected and washed for re-use by the street hawkers.

The sellers were usually young men who located themselves in various parts of the city, generally near the market places. They were given a short course on how to sell their medicines before beginning the job. The bottles were placed on a cloth spread upon the ground or sidewalk. Beside the medicine bottles a typed list framed in glass indicated the medicines being sold and the types of illness or difficulties they could cure. Most of the medicines were liquids which came in attractive pastel shades of color, but a few bottles contained powder. All the medicines cost the same price: two shillings and fifty cents.

The following list of fifteen medicines was copied from the frame list of a Magomeni hawker. The English translations and notes in parentheses are my own:

1. *Kiserewa: Kuruka matego* (lit. to jump traps, e.g. to avoid/ cure sorcery): *moyo* (heart); *kujifungua uzazi* (to make a woman bear children).

2. *Albaini Kamili: kutapisha uchawi* (to vomit uchawi); *nyoka* (snake bite); *jino* (toothache); *sikio* (earache).

3. *Mkashali: kuongeza nguvu ya kiume* (to increase the sexual potency of a man).

4. *Gumbo: ngiri* (hernia); *gonolia* (gonorrhea).

5. *Rukago: zindiko la nyumba inayoingiwa na wachawi* (for protection of a house vulnerable to witches).

6. *Kazania: kuhara damu* (dysentery); *mama anatumika zaidi* (to stop abnormal menstrual bleeding).

7. *Kasanyinyi: upele* (scabies); *jipu* (boils); *jino* (toothache).

8. *Rafa: macho giza* (lit. eye darkness, for failing eyesight); *macho gere* (eye illness).

9. *Kanene: kutoa mapembe mabaya nyumbani yanayo pulu watu* (to remove bad horns from the house which harm people. Horns here refers to bad medicine used for sorcery).

10. *Paramanatis: tetekuwanga* (chicken pox); *ndui* (smallpox); *jipu* (boils).

11. *Mayati: surua* (measles); *yabisi* (rheumatism).

12. *Kapitani: kifua* (chest colds); *tibii* (tuberculosis); *pumu* (lung asthma); *kifadulo* (whooping cough).

13. *Kangazi: kutoa michango tumboni* (to remove worms or stomach diseases).

14. *Dombora: kutombo* (abnormally large stomach); *kimeo* (throat - lit. little tongue); *kifafa* (epilepsy); *degedege la mtoto* (lit. - when a bird has frightened a child - convulsions).

15. *Chogo: kutoa muksi mwilini* (to remove the bad smell/spirit from the body).

If the healing powers accredited to these fifteen medicines did work as advertised, then the scientific medical world had indeed a great deal to learn from the company of African Native Medicines and its promoters. But, when the same bottle of medicine could cure measles or rheumatism, epilepsy or throat trouble, hernia or gonorrhea, then one might begin to question this colored and perfumed water, selling for two shillings and fifty cents a bottle.

One seller stated that "People from the country buy these medicine bottles when they come to the market to sell their fruit and other food stuffs." There is no doubt that the ten to twelve street medicine sellers had a growing trade, and the city license bureau and Ministry of Health had not questioned the honesty of such medicine. If in fact people using No. 12 - *Kapitani* were cured of tuberculosis and lung asthma, it would seem advisable for the Ministry of Health to investigate the properties of such medicine.

5. Muwizi, Circumcisers

I have added the *muwizi*, circumcisers, to the list of medical practitioners, because in a very real sense they perform a medical function among the Zaramo. It must be said that circumcisers are not called waganga by the local society. Two *muwizi* interviewed stressed very strongly that medicine men treat people for illness of different sorts but a *muwizi* treats only those whom he circumcises. I include the *muwizi* in this study of the medicine men because their practice is widespread and if it were not performed by the *muwizi* it would most certainly be performed in hospitals by medical doctors.

In search for medicine men in Dar es Salaam three *muwizi* were discovered, two in Buguruni and one in Ilala. No doubt there are many more in the city but, because they do not use the title of mganga, they were not discovered in this survey. The three circumcisers located were all Muslim Zaramo men. *Jando* or *kumbi*, circumcision camps, where these men function, are located in the bush land just outside Dar es Salaam's residential areas of Kinondoni, Buguruni, Kigogo, Yombo, Tandika and Ubungo. The boys' initiation camps are held each year at these locations, during which time the circumcision takes place. The *muwizi* may also be called upon to perform the operation privately in the client's home. This service is more profitable for the *muwizi* and is a growing practice in Dar es Salaam.

The *muwizi* stated that they were not waganga but that they knew several types of medicine connected with this work. Special medicine is used for healing the circumcision wound, and medicines for cases of infection must be known. In this study of the waganga the *muwizi* were the only persons who performed surgical operations. In the normal traditional medical practice the waganga may in some instances make small incisions on the body in order to rub in powdered medicine, but to my knowledge the *muwizi* performs the only surgical operation.

The *muwizi* informants said that they must also know a degree of *uchawi* and protection medicine against sorcery. They said that because of rivalry at the *jando* camp the *muwizi* try to "bewitch" each other, thus necessitating knowledge of medicines for protection.

The *jando* camps are neither organized nor operated by the *muwizi* but rather by men called *Mkema Kumbi*. Parents wishing their boys to be circumcised contact the Mkema Kumbi. All parents must provide a *kungwi*, guardian, to look after their boy and to assist in feeding and instructing him. The Mkema Kumbi who runs the camp employs the *muwizi*, who not only circumcises the boys but also helps instruct them in the initiation songs. The *muwizi* is paid a fee of approximately 10 shillings by each parent whose son is to be circumcised.

As every Zaramo male is circumcised, this is a notable ongoing business for traditional *muwizi* circumcisers. Even though there is a trend these days towards hospital circumcisions, this accounts for only 11 per cent of the boys according to my survey. *Muwizi* will therefore continue to have a substantial practice for some time to come. According to the birth rate of the Zaramo population, well over 1,000 Zaramo boys from Dar es Salaam are circumcised each year. The majority of the boys are sent to camps in "home" villages. As the city population grows, so will the local numbers increase in the six camp locations in the Dar es Salaam area.

I have not included the *muwizi* in any of the statistical analyses given in this study, nor have I included them when discussing the work of the traditional waganga. It is important, however, that we recognize the work of the circumcisers who perform this surgical operation and who in their own practice demonstrate an appropriate amount of medical knowledge.

6. Midwives

It is noted in Dar es Salaam that a growing number of Zaramo give birth to their children in hospitals and clinics. Sixty-five per cent of the Zaramo said their children were born or will be born in a hospital or clinic. This still leaves a sizeable number who give birth to their children at home and who are assisted by local traditional midwives.

Again, as in the case of *muwizi*, circumcisers, the *wazalishi*, Sw., midwives, perform a medical function but are never referred to as waganga in the traditional sense. As the number of prenatal clinics and maternity hospitals increases, the number of births in homes will decrease. This will in turn lessen the need for traditional midwives. Health education given in school and in medical clinics tends to discourage home deliveries.

I never heard of Zaramo midwives who sold their services in the same way as *muwizi*, circumcisers. The midwife is simply a mother or grandmother in the local area who has acquired enough experience and knowledge over the years to be of assistance during the time of delivery. Usually she is a kin or clan member who is called upon for this help.

NOTES TO CHAPTER 2

[1]For additional information on witch eradication movements in Eastern Africa, see: Douglas, Mary, "Techniques of Sorcery Control", in Middleton, J. and Winter, E.H. (eds.), *Witchcraft and sorcery in East Africa*. London: Routledge and Kegan Paul, 1963, 123-142; Willis, R.G., "The Kamcape Movement", in Marwick, M. (ed.), *Witchcraft and Sorcery*. Harmondsworth: Penguin, 1970, 184-198.

[2]In 1972 sixty cents in Tanzanian money equaled approximately 8 cents U.S. currency: 100 cents = 1 shilling: 7 shillings= US$ 1.00.

[3]Referring to their light skin: also Indians or light-skinned Arabs can thus be referred to as Wazungu.

CHAPTER 3
Diagnosis of Illness - the Diviner

In Swahili there are several word forms used to designate a diviner and divination. *Mwaguzi*, Sw. means diviner, coming from the Swahili verb *ku-agua*, to see, to divine, predict, prophesy. More often, the words *mpiga ramli* or *mpiga bao* are used to designate the one who divines. *Ramal*, Ar., *ramli*, Sw., means divination, as well as the less common words *uramli*, *uaguzi* and *ubashiri*.

The Zaramo forms for diviner and divination have almost entirely been replaced in conversation by Swahili words. *Ku-lagula* is the Zaramo verb to divine and *ndagu*, Z., the word for divination. These are seldom used today. In earlier times the Zaramo differentiated between the types of *ndagu*: e.g. *ndagu ya kifo*, divination for death; *ndagu ya ugonjwa*, divination for sickness; *ndagu ya safari*, divination for travel or hunting; *ndagu ya vita*, divination for war; or *ndagu ya uchuro*, divination for omens of events (Mwaruka, 1965, 80 ff.). Today these distinctions between the types of divining or diviners are seldom made. Zaramo simply speak about going to a mganga, medicine man, for almost all diviners are medicine men. The Swahili expression *kwenda kutuzama*, "to go to look," is also used very often when referring to divination.

1. The Role of the Diviner

The Zaramo living in Dar es Salaam have several possible ways of finding out the cause of their illness or misfortune or a death in the family. If they have bodily illness there is the option of going to a government hospital or clinic where the diagnosis will be made on the basis of laboratory tests; symptoms and observations, or they may choose to go to a traditional diviner who will use one of several methods to discern the nature of the disease, its cause, and a method of cure. They may also choose to go to a Muslim *shehe* or *mwalimu*, whose ability in divination is particularly respected.

A Zaramo may go first to a government hospital for the cure of the illness or the setting of a broken bone, but will then proceed to the diviner to find out who caused this trouble and how it can be avoided in the future. The basic question for most of the Zaramo is not "What is the illness I have?" but rather, "Who has made it happen to me and what shall I take or do for protection?" Very often, as we shall see in the case studies, patients in the hospital feel that they are recovering too slowly or not at all, and therefore send a relative to a diviner to find out if the real problem has been caused by sorcery which "European medicine" cannot cure. If so, they may leave the hospital and go to a mganga.

Diviners hold a key position in the traditional medical system, for it is they who determine whether the client has been bewitched or poisoned, has broken a taboo, dishonored ancestor spirits, or whether he or she has tuberculosis and should visit a government doctor. The findings of diviners are believed and followed without question. What they reveal through their divination is believed to be absolute fact for the majority of Zaramo. Diviners have the respect and confidence of the people. They play the role of counsellor, fortune teller and revealer of secrets. By their judgments revealing the causes of illness they become the preservers of traditional Zaramo customs and religious practices.

The diviners' work deals with both private and public affairs. They may recommend to a football team that they cancel a scheduled match if the omens show that they will lose that day. They decide the day and hour to begin the dance for the coming-out rites of a *mwali*, young girl, or when to begin the initiation, *jando*, camp or when to hold an exorcism *madogoli*. Diviners are called in to determine whether or not two people should get married. They may recommend that the girl not take a new name because her present one has greater "value" than the name of her future husband. The Zaramo invariably see in every death an intervention by hostile forces, usually the work of sorcery, and this must be verified. Again, it is the task of a diviner to explain the problem.

It should be stated that whereas all diviners are waganga, not all waganga practise divining. Either they did not inherit the gift or learn the art, or they do not believe in this method of diagnosis of problems. Seven of the 38 questioned indicated that they do not divine. This question was not administered systematically to every mganga interviewed in my study and therefore is based on a smaller sample of waganga. Nevertheless, it is a fair assumption to believe that no fewer than three-quarters of the waganga in Dar es Salaam can conduct some form of divination.

In addition to the divining practised by traditional medicine men, the Muslim *shehe* and *mwalimu* play a major role as diviners. All *washehe* and *mwalimu* perform some acts which can be termed divination, as well as practising some forms of healing. The art of divining is part of the training given to all Muslim *shehe* and *mwalimu*, and special books are used for the system based on geomancy (numbers). The term used to describe this form of divining in Swahili is *ramli ya kitabu*, divination of the book, and their form of medicine is called *dawa ya kitabu*, medicine of the book. This Muslim form of book divining is not limited to use by the *shehe* and *mwalimu*; a large number of traditional medicine men with a smattering of Koranic training have adapted it in various ways. There is no apparent competition between Muslim diviners and traditional diviners. Each, of course, is looking for customers and will indirectly indicate that he is willing to take on the person as a client. It is not uncommon, however, for a *shehe* or *mwalimu* to send the client to a traditional mganga for the cure. The general practice is that one mganga or Muslim *shehe* or *mwalimu* will do the divining and another will give the medicine for cure or protection. In the analysis of 100 cases we shall see the statistics on the actual practice.

How do you become a diviner? This question relates very closely to the question of how you become a mganga. From the interviews with waganga, this appeared to be one and the same question. The large number of traditional diviners answering this question used the Muslim *kitabu* method and therefore had gone to Koran school as children. In their youth or adulthood they had studied under a *mwalimu* tutor or mganga using the *kitabu* method. Seven of the twelve using the *kitabu* method used the title of *mwalimu*, indicating that they had had Islamic training in divining, but they were not teaching children in Koran school, leading prayers or teaching the Koran. For them *Mwalimu* was used as a prestige title and would indicate to prospective clients that they perform *ramli* and *uganga* according to the book. The second largest group using variations of the *bao*, the board method, learned the art from other diviners. It is common to work several years as an apprentice under an experienced medicine man. Some said they had studied under several waganga. As the mganga gains experience he develops his own technique of *ramli* and may vary or add to what he has learned from others.

Those who use the *Rungu manyanga* or *mbizi* method must first be possessed by the Rungu spirit. This spirit may force the person through illness or possession to become a diviner and mganga. The Rungu spirit and Rungu *uganga* may also be inherited. In this case the expression "inherit the bag," *mfuko*, Sw., is used. The bag may be inherited from either parents or grandparents after their death. Some who may have learned *ramli* and *uganga* from their parents will then practise the trade immediately, but more often, even if they have *mfuko*, they will undergo an apprenticeship with a mganga of their particular spirit.

Divining is not the monopoly of any one ethnic group in Dar es Salaam. The numbers correspond fairly closely to the ratio of each ethnic group represented in the city and to the number of waganga from each.

2. Methods of Divining Used in Dar es Salaam

I asked a total of 45 diviners about their methods of divining. Of these 36 were traditional diviners and 9 were Muslim *shehe* and *mwalimu*. All 9 *shehe* and *mwalimu* used the *kitabu* book method, and so did 9 of the traditional diviners. Other methods used by the traditional diviners were the *bao* board (7), the Rungu spirit (8), *kitabu* and *bao* together (2), *kitabu* and gourd with beads and powder (1), Rungu and dreams (1). Eight traditional diviners did not reveal their method. It should be noted that some diviners can use two methods and that within each general method there are variations and novelties in practice. Some descriptions of divining as observed in Dar es Salaam now follow.

a. Spirit Divining - Rungu Ramli

Divining with the help of particular spirits is one of the most common forms used by the Zaramo, Kwere, Kutu, and Zigua ethnic groups on the coast. The Rungu spirit diviners are more numerous than those who divine with the help of Kinyamkera, Mwenembago or Kilinge spirits.

The Rungu (or Lungu, pl. Malungu, Marungu) spirit is often referred to as the spirit of a snake and is connected with the Kolelo shrine in the Uluguru Mountains. Rungu is said to have a snake or a lion as his servant and the spirit appears in these forms during the exorcism rites. Rungu divining and the Rungu exorcism rites are practised by waganga who have the *jadi* of Rungu and who themselves have been possessed by the Rungu spirit. The Rungu spirit is said to give the diviner power to "see." Whether this "seeing" is extra-sensory perception, intuitive knowledge, hypnotic suggestion or plain common sense is difficult to determine. The Rungu diviners say they do not see as in a dream or trance, but that the information "just comes" to them when they sing. Nine diviners in the survey listed Rungu Ramli as their method of divining.

Mganga A.S., a Zaramo medicine man living in Kariakoo, was a typical "Rungu divining" mganga. A.S. was about 50 years old at the time of the study. He was a Muslim and had two wives. He owned a house and a *shamba*, farm, in the country near Bunju, and rented a Swahili-type house in Dar es Salaam, where he practised divining and traditional medicine. As a farmer raising cashew-nut trees and rice, Mganga A.S. was no richer or poorer than most farmers in Bunju. He was a leader in the community, having been elected as a representative for Bunju on The Mzizima District Council. As a medicine man, A.S. showed considerable energy and talent and had a willingness to venture forward in this business. In 1968 he moved to Kariakoo, the older central housing area of Dar es Salaam because, he said, "I can make more money in Dar es Salaam doing *uganga* there." He went back to Bunju periodically to look after his *shamba* and to take care of his clients living there, as well as to collect new supplies of roots, grass and herbs as needed for his *uganga.*

Mganga A.S. became a Rungu diviner and mganga through being possessed by this spirit, remaining mentally ill for two years. His relatives thought he was bewitched, which is usually considered the main cause of mental illness. He was taken to *waganga wa kitabu*, medicine men of the book, because they have the power to cause madness and also to cure it. A.S. was taken to three waganga: one in Dar es Salaam, one in Bunju and one in Mlingotini, but none could cure him. He bought two goats, *doti ya bafta*, two lengths of white cloth and all other required items, but nothing helped. He was exorcised for the Kinyamkera spirit through a *madogoli*, but that was no help. He claimed that he and his relatives spent 1,575 shillings on medicine and medicine men, but found no cure. "Then I knew I had to be *pungwa*, exorcised for the Rungu spirit," said Mganga A.S. "The *shetani*, spirit, told this through me." He was taken to a Rungu mganga near Bunju, where he was exorcised and became well. "From that time on I had to do this work. I do not like it, but I got my health back because of it."

According to Mganga A.S., his mother's mother was a mganga of the spirit Kinyamkera and he inherited his *mfuko*, medicine bag, of Kinyamkera from her. He was exorcised and initiated into the Kinyamkera cult at the time of his two-year illness, but he divined and exorcised only by the Rungu method. Mganga A.S. stated that he did not get Rungu directly from either side of his family except that "It is there at the *chamguko cha asili*, source of his ancestry of both families."

Rungu divination sessions were performed by Mganga A.S. in the following manner. After the initial formalities, the client sat on a mat on the floor before the mganga and one or more of his assistants. The mganga himself sat on a wooden stool. The assistants could be apprentices, friends or his wife, who also had the Rungu spirit. They could even be clients living with the mganga while undergoing treatment, as in the case of those observed with Mganga A.S. During the session the assistant interpreted the message of the mganga to the client. Mganga A.S. and the assistants began by the rhythmic shaking of the *mbizi* or *manyanga* wooden rattles (14 centimeters in length) to which three bells were attached at the center. While they all shook their rattles the mganga began his first song. He called upon the names of the Rungu spirits and their dwelling places: Kolelo, Mhanga Lugome, Kibamanduka. He sometimes sang the names of the waganga living and dead through which the spirit had come down to him. As he sang his main message, the assistants sang the refrain in chorus. After the first song the client paid his initial fee of 50 cents and then the singing and rattles continued.

The diviner sang songs mainly used in exorcism rites. These songs included a repetitive stanza which the assistants sang in response. In these often very short songs the mganga began to weave in his message to the client. The diviner closed his eyes as he sang, but did not usually go into a trance. In this singing state he began to "see" the one in need of divining, the problem and the perpetrator of it. The mganga's information began by elimination of the possibilities which had no bearing on the case before him. The client sitting before him might possibly be only an agent for the sick person left in another village. The diviner must discern this fact. The client may be ill, or his problem may be that of theft or bad dreams (sorcery), or it may be a death in the family. These things the diviner must discover, and after ascertaining who is suffering the misfortune he must find out what the client's problem is and what has caused it.

As the mganga sang his thoughts, revealing more and more information, there was a pause after each song. The assistant then translated into Swahili the diviner's message if the client did not understand the mganga's song language, and he gave the client a chance to say whether or not the information revealed was correct. If it was, the client showed his approval by saying "*Tawile*, your words are correct," after which the mganga continued to sing, revealing further information or eliminating that which was not pertinent to the case. This gave the mganga direction as to how he should proceed in the next song. If the diviner did not reveal the case properly, the client would not say "*Tawile*", in which case there was no further payment and the client would go to some other mganga.

Mganga A.S. normally spoke Swahili to his clients and friends in everyday conversation. He spoke Zaramo on some occasions with older Zaramo. But in his songs he used Luguru and Zigua, the languages of his Rungu spirit. A spirit may speak various languages depending on the language abilities of the mganga medium. In this case, Mganga A.S. received his first Rungu exorcism from a Zigua mganga living near Bunju. This may account for his using the Zigua language in the songs, as he probably learned them from this mganga during the time of his illness. The Rungu spirit itself originates from Kolelo in East Luguru, undoubtedly the source of the Luguru songs. It should be stated that both languages are similar to Zaramo and people of these ethnic groups understand each others' language. For those who know only Swahili, or have a limited understanding of Zaramo, the songs must be translated. This is standard procedure for all waganga in Dar es Salaam who use languages other than Swahili in divining.

Divination sessions lasted anywhere from half an hour to one hour, continuing until Mganga A.S. had revealed all the information. He believed that the Rungu spirits communicated with him, but when interviewed he could not explain how. He could only say that it was not through a dream. At times the mganga might "see" no clear message, in which case he would acknowledge his failure to the client and discontinue the divination session.

Only if the session was completed successfully did the client pay the total fee of three shillings. The mganga was usually willing to take on the client for the cure or protection or whatever had to be done. It is part of the task of the diviner to determine to which waganga the client might go for the cure. The final choice is left to the client, but if the diviner desires to take on the case he will impress upon the client his own abilities to treat just such matters. At other times he will recommend a specialist known to be skilled in treating the particular problem.

Mganga A.K. was Kwere by tribe and about 45-50 years old. He lived in the Mtoni area of Dar es Salaam but was performing *ramli* in the Tandika area of Temeke when visited for *ramli* by my assistant. Mganga A.K. divined by the Rungu spirit method using rattles and singing as outlined in the previous case.

Several years before this session, my Zaramo assistant had a motorcycle accident which resulted in a broken arm / shoulder bone. The bone had not been set properly and had since then been giving him trouble. The medical doctor at the hospital told him it must be broken again and reset in order to mend properly and stop hurting. The assistant considered this as his problem when he went to Mganga A.K. for divining. The following account is from my assistant's case notes:

> I asked him if he could try to see what was wrong with my right arm. Then he started playing the rattles. After two introductory songs he started telling me by singing that I am having a very good job and I am very well paid. (Note: He was wearing a white shirt that day), and that I'm a very wealthy person. (Note: His pay was that of a primary school teacher: he is in no sense wealthy.) My neighbor and my co-workers do not like it, so some have bewitched me. (Note: The mganga was careful to include both neighbors and co-workers. This excludes very few people.) He went on saying that the arm won't be cured unless I undergo a very big treatment. . . that I have to find a mganga who really knows about this kind of sorcery. If I don't do it very soon my arm won't be able to work and I will be unable to write. This is how my enemies want it. They want me to fail at work so that I become poor. He went on saying: "My friend, the people are very much against you, take a good step on your arm as soon as possible. You must get a mganga who can *kinga*, protect you."

The *ramli* songs continued for about fifty minutes. During this time the mganga tried to convince him that he really knew how to treat such cases and could get him out of the trouble. He tried indirectly to persuade him to chose Mganga A.K. for the treatment. The charge for the *ramli* was 2 shillings. The mganga did not reveal that the bone was broken in a motorcycle accident and that it had been set poorly. The assistant was still bothered with the arm two years later, but could still write and had a comparatively good job.

The diviner in this case read into the life of the client a situation where supposed jealousy over his job and wealth caused a neighbor or co-worker to bewitch him and cause pain in his arm. Most clients would have paid up to 200 shillings for a cure of the pain and protection from sorcery. If the word of the diviner had been taken seriously it might have resulted in suspicion and accusations at work or the client's moving from his lodgings because of fear of further bewitching by neighbors.

b. Bao Divining

Bao, Sw. (a board). It is also the name of a popular African game played by moving seeds, shells or stones in holes carved into a rectangular board. *Bao*, when used with the verb *ku-piga*, Sw. to strike, beat, hit, means to divine or take omens with the use of a divining board. The divining board may be of plain wood or it may have lines drawn on it, with various numbers or symbols drawn in the squares. Sometimes sand is spread over a board on which lines are drawn. The *bao* board today need not be made of wood, but may be a cloth or a mat with similar lines or no lines. *Bao* may also refer to divining on sand or soil on the ground onto which corn, beads, pebbles, bones or other objects are rolled as would be done also on the wooden board or cloth.

Bao divining, as observed in Dar es Salaam, is often mixed with Islamic geomancy methods of divining. The following examples from interviews with Dar es Salaam diviners will illustrate these variations.

Mganga S.S. was a Zaramo Muslim living in the Buguruni area. He came to Dar es Salaam as a boy and was about 35 years old. He had had Koran training and therefore used both the titles *mwalimu* and mganga. He did not, however, teach children or adults or take part in any mosque or Muslim functions. His title *mwalimu* only added to his status. Mganga S.S. was well-known in the Buguruni-Ilala area. On three different visitations he had more than fifteen clients each time waiting outside for consultation. It was said that many government workers at the Ilala *Boma*, regional headquarters, consulted Mganga S.S. to deal with their sorcery problems.

Anyone wanting to see Mganga S.S. had to wait his turn on the benches and mats in the courtyard behind the house and in the hallway of the Swahili-type house. Before entering, the client removed his shoes and then sat on a mat before the mganga, who was seated on a large pillow on the mat. He was surrounded by a collection of various roots and herbs and colored papers: red, blue and orange. On a table to the side, bottles containing fluids of various colors were arranged. The Koran and other Muslim books were placed beside him. He divined and practised *uganga* between 7 a.m. and 12 o'clock noon, and again from 2 p.m. until late evening. He explained: "From 12 noon until 2 p.m. I cannot see anything . . . They are bad hours."

After the exchange of greetings and hearing the request for *ramali*, the mganga placed on the mat in front of the client a handful of maize kernels. He asked the client to choose any kernel he wished while he himself left the room chanting verses from the Koran. When he returned he started to arrange the kernels in different ways on the mat until he located the one which the client had secretly chosen. Following this he continued chanting in Arabic more verses of the Koran, observing the arrangement of the maize kernels on the mat. After consulting the *Satrikhabari*, he told his client what his trouble was and how he should proceed to solve it.

Mganga S.S. charged 3 shillings for divining, but for any type of treatment it was never less than 40 shillings. People who suffered from mental disturbances had to pay up to 200 shillings for treatment. It was said that if clients did not give him enough money "to make him happy" he might make them suffer again. Mganga S.S. was very finely dressed, and from the appearance of his house seemed a comparatively wealthy man.

Diviner/Mganga S.N. used a combination of *bao* and book divining, and charged 3 shillings for his services. After the usual greeting between the diviner and his client the mganga took ten or more *vizumna*, small cowrie-like shells, on which numbers were written. He put these shells into a small bag of white cloth and shook them three times, at the same time chanting words from the Koran. He gave the bag to his client and asked him to repeat his words as he shook the bag and as the mganga twisted a cloth around both of the client's arms.

Taking a wooden tray with eight holes carved into it, similar to a *bao* board game, the mganga asked the client to shake the shells into the tray. The mganga picked up the shells and asked the client's name or the name of the person who needed this divining. If the name had 4, 5, 6 or more letters, he took shells which followed the number of the letters. He also divined the other shells and subtracted the numbers according to his system. The result of all this was evaluated according to the rules in his *Satrikhabari* book. Also included in his evaluation was the month, day and hour the client came to see him.

After his evaluation was made according to his book, the mganga/diviner told the client what his trouble was and what should be taken for the cure. In this case we see both the traditional method with shells and board being used together with incantations from the Koran and the Islamic geomancy system used according to the *Satrikhabari*.

Mganga B. 212 divined by making drawings in the sand while chanting in the Ngoni language. An assistant translated it into Swahili for the client. Mganga B.216, a Swahili, also made drawings on the ground while divining.

Mganga K. 12, a Zaramo, divined with seeds, which he kept in a *kibuyu* gourd. The seeds popped out of the gourd on their own, without the mganga's help. Depending on which seeds popped out of the gourd, the mganga could divine the case. Divining through the means of dreams and divining with colored powders and a gourd were other methods found in Dar es Salaam.

Mganga A.K. lived in Ilala. He was a Zaramo Muslim whose father and father's father were also medicine men. He was keeper of Kinyamkera *mzimu* spirit hut, built under a *mwale*, raphia palm tree, in Masaki, 40 miles southwest of Dar es Salaam. Once a year he went to Masaki to clean the spirit hut and make his ritual offering, but during the rest of the year this *mzimu* helped him divine through dreams.

When a client went to Mganga A.K. for *ramli*, he directed him or her to go home and return the next morning. During the night the mganga would dream. He claimed that his *mzimu* told him in the night what was wrong with the client and what to do. If he was told that the client had sickness, he was advised in the dream what medicine to make. Mganga A.K. insisted that his *uganga* was not guesswork, but that he had first to be told what to do in his dreams.

Mganga M.C. knew two kinds of divining, *uaguaji*, Sw., but he did not use them both at the same time. He knew how to divine with the book, using the Koran and the book *Satrikhabari*, or he could divine with the use of *usembe*, colored powders, and *tumba*, Sw. gourd. He charged 4 shillings for either kind of *ramli*.

When confronted with a client, Mganga M.C. first considered which of the two divining methods he should use. If it was the *usembe-tumba* method he continued in this way. First he gave the client *usembe*, a powder substance, in three colors - white, red and brown (the color of dry leaves). He offered it with his left hand and the client received it in his own left hand. Then he gave the client a piece of a broken pot and asked him to mix the three colors of *usembe* together on it. At this point Mganga M.C. would begin to chant, revealing the reason for the client's visit. The mganga put the *usembe* into a gourd which had white, black and red beads on its neck and covered the gourd with a cloth for five to ten minutes. When he opened the top of the gourd and asked it (the gourd) what his client had come for, the gourd gave the answers. It was not a voice speaking understandable words, but sounded like "*korowanga-korowanga.*" The mganga would understand the meaning of the sound and translate it to the client, thus disclosing what was troubling him, and the cause of it. If the *tumba*, gourd, did not succeed in explaining the difficulty satisfactorily, it admitted the failure itself. The gourd might say, "Today I do not see well; for this reason go to another diviner." The mganga would translate this to the client.

When asked the reason for using two methods of divining - the book and the gourd - the diviner explained, "The *wachawi*, sorcerers, are very clever in their ways of bewitching and hiding themselves, because after they bewitch they bathe with medicines called *kiziza*. They bathe with these medicines in a pit, a *umolelanga*, Z. in the earth, or at the crossroads at night, or beside a running river. You cannot find these *wachawi* when divining with a book. It is necessary to use the *kishenzi*, Sw. pagan way, of divining for finding pagan sorcerers, so I use the *tumba*, gourd. This is the reason I have learned to divine both ways."

After relating the above information, Mganga M.C. began scratching his stomach. When he pulled up his shirt to scratch better, three *hirizi*, amulets, were seen tied about his waist. My assistant joked, saying, "Look, you my friend have all you need, you don't need to fear sorcerers." The mganga replied, "Sorcerers hate us waganga because we save people whom they have bewitched in order to kill. When they see that many get well, they take counsel to bewitch and kill us so that we are out of the way. This is the reason why you have to strengthen yourself first before you can cure others."

c. Ramli ya kitabu - Book Divining

The method of divining used by the largest group of traditional medicine men in Dar es Salaam is the Islamic form of geomancy. This method employs incantations from the Koran as well as making calculations and evaluations of each case from a book known as *Satrikhabari* by the local people. More than one third of all medicine men questioned as to the method they use specified the *kitabu* method. In addition to the traditional medicine men, all the *washehe* and *walimu*, Muslim clerics and Koran teachers, said they use the *kitabu* method of divining.

It seems that all Islamic diviners in Dar es Salaam have studied the book called *Satrikhabari*, Sw. and use it in their practise. The study of divining and *uganga* according to Islamic forms is often referred to as the study of *elimu ya dunia*, education of the world. This training is acquired in formal Muslim training centers at Bagomoyo, Kilwa, Kivinje and Zanzibar. Since the union between Zanzibar and Tanganyika mainland, travel between these two areas has had more restrictions, so fewer students from the mainland go to Zanzibar to study. The same training is more often received by studying independently under a *shehe*, *mwalimu* or mganga who has himself acquired the knowledge and is willing to teach it to others. Besides the *Satrikhabari*, the book *Abu Ma'shar al-Falaki* and the treatise of Muhammad az-Zanati, *Kitab al-fasl fi usul 'ilm ar-raml* are also said to be used in the coastal area. (Swantz, M-L. 1970, 128; Trimingham, 1964, 124.) None of these, however, were mentioned by informants on *ramli* in Dar es Salaam.

Liturgical incantations from the Koran are often read during the divination session. The main *sura*, chapters, used are 1, *Fatiha*, Ar., 113, *Al-Falaq*, Ar. - "The Daybreak" and 114, *An-nas*, Ar. "Mankind." Portions of *Hal Badri* (*Ahl al Badr*, Ar., *Halubadili*, Sw.) and *Dala 'ilal Khairat* and *Burdat* are used in connection with the treatment following the *ramli*.

In the eyes of many local Zaramo who cannot read or write, the mystery and power associated with a book is very attractive. The knowledge of astrology and the mystery of symbols and numbers written in Arabic with chalk on a plate look very impressive. The following cases are samples of different forms of Islamic divining in Dar es Salaam as recorded from interviews with waganga and Muslim clerics.

Mganga C. was well known throughout Dar es Salaam and according to all reports and our own reports and our own interviews with him, had perhaps the largest traditional practice of uganga in the city. He had three assistants helping him, one of whom was a fully-fledged mganga who could take over whenever the chief, Mganga C., was not present. Mganga C. was Makua by tribe and received his *uganga* from his father, who was a traditional mganga as well as a Koran teacher. My assistant called him both *mwalimu* and mganga. As Mganga C. led no prayers nor taught the Koran, I have not considered him as a Muslim cleric in this study. The "*Mwalimu* " title was not used by Mganga C. himself, nor by my second assistant who interviewed him on two other occasions. Mganga C. used only the Islamic form of divining, while his medicine and form of treatment was either that of the book or of herbs. The majority of the clients who came to him were Zaramo.

When a client came to him, the mganga began by noting the day, month and hour. Then he asked the name of the person for whom the divining was to be done. Since it was not necessary for the troubled individual to be present in person, a friend or relative would often go to the diviner on his or her behalf. After hearing the name of the client, the diviner asked also the name of the client's father. These names were written with chalk on a slate and the letters in each word were counted and numbers given to each according to the number values of the letters. Having done this he subtracted the numbers from each other by a method which he would not disclose. He then took his book of *ramli*, *Satrikhabari*, and compared the number with the time of the client's visit as well as with the type of weather outside. After this he could explain to the person what the trouble was that brought the client to him, whether it was a matter of sorcery, theft, sickness, or a broken taboo. Finally, he looked for the medicines which were prescribed in the book.

As an explanation for the writing of numbers, the mganga said it meant *Kuvuta jumu*, to draw stars. (*Jumu*, star, as an omen, often an ill omen.)He also commented that every man has his own stars of luck, and life must be looked at carefully when divining through these.

Mwalimu A.S. was a Zaramo of Kariakoo. When clients went to Mwalimu A.S. they were not asked for their names. He took hold of the client's left hand and said, "Let all your secret words (matters) be raised up, *inuliza maneno yako yote komoyomoyo* " - meaning the trouble which brought the person for treatment. He then started looking at his book (*Satrikhabari*). He noted the day, the time, the weather, sun, clouds, or rain. When he finished reading he immediately began to reveal the client's problem, with such examples as: "I see this person who is ill; he is not far from me; he is a man, black and tall." If the client agreed that what he said was correct, she responded by saying "*Tawile* ", meaning "It is correct." The *mwalimu* continued by revealing more and more about the trouble which brought the client to him. When the divining was completed, the client had to decide whether she wanted this *mwalimu* to handle the case or whether she preferred to take her case to another mganga. If she wished the diviner to continue with the case she would say, "*Kiguzo* ", meaning "Support or comfort me, you are the mganga."

If the client wanted another mganga to take on her or his case then Mwalimu A.S. divined again to determine who the mganga should be. This second divination was not done with the book but by the *bao* board method, to see whether the medicine which was needed was his or whether it belonged to some other mganga. He asked the client to mention the name of another mganga. The client continued to mention names of different waganga until the diviner "saw" by the way the beads were thrown on the board that the client would have good luck with him. The client would then go to this mganga designated through divination and would tell him everything he or she had learned from the diviner.

Mwalimu A.S. collected two shillings from everyone who came to him for divining. He asked those who gave the money to put it under the prayer mat near his incense burner.

Mganga N.S.K. was an elderly Zaramo who came to Dar es Salaam long ago from the Bagamoyo area. He was well known in the city for helping clients with court cases, as well as those who wanted to keep their jobs or avoid transfers. Mganga N.S.K. used a combination of book divining and scissors as his rather distinct form of *ramli*.

When first meeting his client there was an exchange of greetings and an enquiry as to the purpose of the visit. If the reply was "*Nimekuja kupiga bao*, I have come for divination," the mganga took out the book *Satrikhabari* but did not open it. He began to chant *sura*, chapters, from the Koran very slowly, instructing the client to take hold of the book three times and to say in his heart secretly the troubles which had brought him to the mganga. Then the mganga took a pair of scissors and pressed them into the corner of the book. While holding the scissors vertically he balanced the book on the point and turned it around many times while chanting words of the Koran. People were amazed that the book did not fall from the tips of the scissor blades.

Following this balancing act, Mganga N.S.K. would open the book and begin to tell the client on whose behalf he had come, whether it was his own trouble or that of his wife or child or relative. He proceeded to tell him whether it was for sickness, sorcery, death, unemployment or some other problem. Following this he told the client what steps should be taken to rid himself of the trouble. The fee for this information was four shillings.

If Mganga N.S.K. was requested by the client to take on the case he would proceed immediately to prepare medicine or take other measures to handle the problem. If this was not desired, the client paid the four shillings and sought another mganga for the treatment.

Because of the apparent success of this mganga, many clients went to him each day. Indians, Goans and Arabs were also said to be among his clients which, in local Zaramo eyes, was proof that he must be very good.

Unlike other Islamic diviners, Mganga N.S.K. did not ask the client for the number of letters in his name, nor did he take obvious notice of the time of the visit and the weather conditions. Furthermore, he did not make the usual mathematical calculations with chalk on a slate. It was said by one informant that the very best diviners need not open their *Satrikhabari* book, as they have it all memorized. Such knowledgeable Muslim clerics or waganga could ask for higher fees, as indeed Mganga N.S.K. did. "The others make it their business only to get just their daily bread," concluded the informant. The scissors balancing act no doubt contributed to the fame of this mganga, although it was not quite clear why he did it, other than to impress people with his skill.

Mganga A.B. of Buguruni employed a method involving small squares of paper with numbers written on them. When a client came for divining he or she was given a handful of these papers and instructed to throw them up in the air, letting them fall down on the mat at random. Then the client was asked to pick them up one by one and hand them to the mganga, who divided them into two piles while looking very carefully at the numbers written on the papers. This act of throwing up the papers, collecting and dividing them into piles, was repeated seven times. After the seventh collection and division of numbers, the mganga wrote his calculations down on his slate and then opened his *Satrikhabari* book to find the meaning. Mganga A.B. also considered in his calculations the month, week, day and hour, as well as the weather. Based on this information the mganga revealed to the client the matters concerning his problem.

The paper-throwing method in the initial stage has some resemblance to throwing bones, seeds or stones, as in the traditional *bao ramli* forms of divination. However, the numbers of the papers and the calculations made follow the more established Islamic geomancy practice.

As can be noted from these twelve forms of *ramli* described above, no two are exactly alike. If twelve more were listed, there would again be variations and a few novelties according to the talents of the practitioners. The mystery and seeming accuracy of the revelations is convincing to most clients. The credibility of the profession rests on the accuracy of the diviner. There is every indication that this is a flourishing business and will continue for some time to come. The following material provides quantitative information on the use of *ramli* by the 100 Zaramo clients interviewed for this study.

3. Frequency of Ramli Divining

Of the 100 clients of waganga, 54 were women and 41 were men; 3 were husband and wife units coming together with the same problem, and 2 cases involved small children brought by their mothers. It may be noted that there are slightly more women going to waganga than men. This is explained by the fact that men working in offices, government employment or factories must report to a government hospital and obtain a doctor's certificate whenever they are ill, otherwise they lose their salary for the days absent from work. In view of this it is surprising that the number of men visiting waganga is as high as it is.

Of these 100 cases, 58 had gone for *ramli*, divining; 25 said they did not go for divining, and 17 made no statement regarding it. Of the 58 cases which did have *ramli*, 41 went in person to a diviner, while 17 had relatives go on their behalf. In all such cases it was a relative who went on their behalf, and not a friend. This indicates the close kinship ties among the Zaramo and the responsibility they assume for each other when in need. Of these 17 kin who went for *ramli* on behalf of another, six were husbands who went for their wives, four were brothers, two were sisters, two fathers, one wife, one mother, and one a mother's brother.

Of the 58 cases who had a diagnosis of their problem through divining, 41 chose to receive treatment from the same medicine man who divined the case. The other 17, or nearly 30 per cent, had gone to a diviner first and were treated on the basis of his diagnosis by a second mganga.

Among the 25 cases who said they had not gone for divining were problems which were so obvious there was no need for divining. For example, there were those seeking employment who wanted only to buy an amulet for good luck. There were several court cases and prison sentences in which clients were seeking medicine to help win the case or have the sentence reduced. There were some who believed themselves to be "just sick" and felt no need for *ramli*. A few also did not belive in the possibility of sorcery, so for them there was no need for *ramli*.

The majority of the 17 cases who made no statement on *ramli* were most likely clients who had actually gone to a diviner but who did not report it. My reason for this assumption is based on the problems listed by these 17 clients, 13 of which were accusations of sorcery which normally are determined through divination. The remaining four problems were two cases of spirit possession, one case of an impending court trial and one case of sickness due to involvement in a murder. These last four cases might not have needed a decision from a diviner as the problems were already known to the clients.

From the above information it can be seen that no fewer than two-thirds to three-quarters of all cases treated by medicine men in Dar es Salaam had first been diagnosed by traditional or Islamic methods. This then is not an isolated event in the life of the Zaramo in Dar es Salaam but must in fact be the object of considerable discussion and activity. It was estimated earlier that, on the basis of the average case load of the 700 waganga in Dar es Salaam, there are approximately 8,000 to 10,000 clients being treated daily. If this is an accurate estimate, then the numbers which are diagnosed by *ramli* methods must run into the thousands each day.

We have seen in this section once again how traditional forms of divination continue in the city, but with variations in style according to the training or preference of the particular diviner. A more radical departure from the traditional Zaramo *bao* and *Rungu* spirit methods of divining has come through the introduction of Islamic forms of *ramli*. More urban diviners today use the Islamic form of geomancy divining than any other single form of traditional divining. In many cases they use two methods, one of them being the Islamic form. Because of the new religious identification with Islam, we clearly see that many diviners have adapted their methods of divination to the forms introduced by Islamic clerics. On the other hand, those who still retain the traditional spirit form of *ramli* can be said to be the preservers of the Zaramo traditional religious concepts.

As a respected seer and prophet, the diviner's diagnosis of illness and misfortune is accepted by the client without question. Because of this unquestioned authority he is in a key position to perpetuate moral, religious and traditional Zaramo concepts and practices. He may credit an illness to the breaking of a clan taboo, the anger of a living-dead ancestor, or the possession of a clan spirit. He may attribute the cause of the misfortune to the work of a witch or sorcerer. In these verdicts he affirms traditional social and religious patterns of belief and practice. We shall see later how the diviner is changing his explanation of the causes of illness and misfortune to suit the new urban situation as well as for his own convenience and that of his client. For example, if he were to attribute the cause to spirit possession or an angered ancestor spirit, the client would need to return to his or her home village for treatment and the diviner would lose his chance to treat the client and therefore the accompanying fee. In contrast to the rural divination cases, we shall see the trend away from accusations against spirits, ancestors, witches and kin members and towards accusations against urban neighbors and co-workers who are said to have used sorcery against the client. Also, because of housing difficulties in the city, it would be difficult for the client to invite all of his or her kin-group to the city to perform a spirit exorcism. The diviner's insight into this problem may lead him to credit the cause of the problem to something he can treat locally on an individual basis. The new urban tensions allow a new set of accusations to be proposed by the diviner, showing adaptation to social change and thus successfully preserving his role in Zaramo society.

CHAPTER 4
The Urban Zaramo and Their Concept of Illness and Misfortune

The information in the preceding sections has generally been descriptive, illustrated with present-day cases. It has been my intention to show what part *uganga* plays in the life pattern and beliefs of the Zaramo. Traditional medicine has been looked at mainly from the point of view and activity of the waganga. Further descriptive material will now illustrate the concept of illness and misfortune from the side of the urban Zaramo client. It will then be possible to determine the role mganga plays in Zaramo life today and the intensity of this activity. We shall ask what it is that attracts the Zaramo to the traditional medicine man today.

First, it is important to get a general picture of the problems which the Zaramo take to the traditional mganga. What areas of Zaramo life are actually touched by the medicine man? Some quantitative information is needed, for "common knowledge" often distorts the facts out of proportion. For example, it may be thought that witches are a critical problem because such news items from court cases have appeared in newspapers and are widely read and talked about. But are the Zaramo of Dar es Salaam troubled by witches? If so, to what degree? Or is their problem that of sorcery or just plain illness, which they feel can be taken care of better by a local mganga than in a hospital or clinic?

I have tried to locate the focus of Zaramo problems treated by the waganga by using three approaches. All three methods contribute valuable evidence to achieve as complete a picture as possible of the actual situation today. I consider the questions and problems now before us as the heart of this study. From this detailed information we can begin to draw the answers and formulate the role of the medicine man as it is today in Dar es Salaam.

The first approach presents evidence from 100 Zaramo cases of illness and misfortune treated by waganga in Dar es Salaam during the field work period. These people were, for the most part, interviewed in the waiting rooms of waganga. Some few were cases being treated by waganga in the client's home and some cases were described by people in homes, bars or on the street after they had been treated by the waganga. All were current or very recent cases.

The second approach used was to ask the waganga to list the various types of problems brought to them, in order of frequency. The third approach was to ask the waganga to list the number of different cases treated the previous day, as well as on the day they were being interviewed. The statistics given on the day the mganga was interviewed are not given in this material because it would be incomplete information; the mganga's work day was generally not over. The question was asked only to see if the mganga's activity and cases were relatively similar to those of the previous day. This appeared to be the case in every instance, so we felt confident that we were receiving accurate information. While sitting in the mganga's waiting room we could also make our own estimate of the cases and numbers of clients. Over a period of fourteen months of such visits we could see consistent patterns and had no reason to disbelieve our informants.

The actual listing of a mganga's case load for a day was a good check on his own estimation of what problems people brought to him. Both sources of information were necessary because it is evident that some information would be missing if only one question was asked. For example, almost all waganga said that politicians and sports teams solicit their help. In the actual case loads of 60 waganga, no help was sought for political problems or difficulties associated with sports. This does not mean that these people do not come, but rather that their problems were not connected with their profession (or it was not an election time or the football season). It must also mean that while most people like to talk about politicians and football players going to the waganga for protection and good luck, in actual practice it must be rather rare. The object in this several-sided exercise was not to determine the exact statistical details for a computerized report, but rather to see the various problems as accurately as possible in the perspective of the total frequency pattern and to determine the causes behind such phenomena. People, their illnesses and social problems and their reasoning processes in understanding their problems are the focal points of the present material.

First, what do the traditional waganga say are the main problems brought to them and how do these compare with the actual combined case load listed for a day?

In this study, 81 traditional waganga were interviewed about their work. Three itinerant waganga coming into Dar es Salaam for witchcraft eradication, but who were fully practising waganga as well, were also interviewed and observed. In addition to these there were 9 Muslim *washehe* and *walimu* practitioners interviewed whose work did not differ greatly from that of the traditional waganga. From this total of 93 practitioners 60 gave details about their previous day's case load as well as answering the questions regarding the types of problems brought to them and the frequency of such cases. The other 33 gave certain amounts of information willingly about their practice, but this was not sufficient in regard to the number of cases treated to be included for statistical purposes with the other 60 waganga.

The various categories of problems brought to waganga for treatment were listed by them as follows:

1. *Ugonjwa*, Sw., Sickness:	This was physical sickness due to sorcery, or physical sickness having no connection with sorcery.
2. *Uchawi*, Sw., Sorcery:	This category may overlap with No. 1, but not always. Death, loss of job, overdue pregnancy, might also be the result of sorcery. The cure of the illness or misfortune might be the first step, but following this the *uchawi* must be removed and the power of the sorcerer counteracted.
3. *Kingwa*, Sw., Protection:	Protection from sorcery as well as from *makungu*, Sw., spirits, *shetani* and *jini* which may or may not be the work of sorcery. *Dawa*, amulets, and the reading of *halubadili* are the main forms of protective treatment given.
4. *Kazi*, Sw., Work:	People come mainly to get jobs, but sometimes it may be to prevent being transferred to another town. This category may overlap with No. 3 for some also come to protect their job so that others at work will not cause them to fail in order to take their position.
5. *Biashara*, Sw., Business:	Mainly to improve and protect their businesses. Shopkeepers, vegetable and fruit sellers and prostitutes seek *dawa* to improve their business and attract new customers.
6. *Shida ya ngono*, Sw., Sexual problems:	This category covers problems of barrenness of women, impotency of men, problems related to sexual taboos and love medicine to attract the opposite sex.
7. *Shida ya ndoa*, Sw., Marriage problems:	This might overlap with No. 6, but is mainly related to marital quarrels, divorce, and problems of unfaithfulness between husband and wife.

8. *Mzimu*, Sw., Spirits and jadi, Sw., Ritual obligations:	This area covers spirit possession and exorcism, neglected spirits, neglected taboos and things concerning the Zaramo *jadi*, ritual obligations.
9. *Mtu mwenye kichaa* or *kwenda wazimu*, Sw., Mental illness:	This problem might overlap with No.1 and 2, for mental illness is always thought to be the work of sorcery. (I have kept it as a separate category for investigation in this study.)
10. *Michezo*, Sw., Sports:	This treatment generally covers protection for the players, good luck medicine to win, and divination to determine what the winning or losing omens are on the day of the game.
11. *Siasa*, Sw., Politics:	This did not come up as one of the major categories listed by waganga but in interviews it was mentioned a number of times and appeared in the cases of the 100 clients.
12. *Kesi za jela* or *Baraza na jela*, Sw., Court and prison cases:	Not a major category, but a few were listed amongst the 100 clients.

The waganga were asked to place in order of frequency the types of cases brought to them, that is, what was first, second, third and so on. This was not a good question, for the waganga were not familiar with statistical arrangements and of course do not keep records or counts of their cases. However, with a little explanation on some occasions, they could understand the question and were able to give their views. This question was also difficult for some to answer because they said some problems came to them in equal numbers. For example, if a person was treated for sorcery, he or she would most certainly return to be treated for protection. Therefore they both might be listed in first place. After a few trial questions we decided to record all those equally numerous for first place with a number "1" and if the mganga said two categories were about equal for second place, they were both listed as number "2". The object of this exercise was simply to gain some understanding of what problems the mganga thought were being brought to him. This, then, could be compared with the actual day's case load given by the mganga as well as to the 100 cases being treated by waganga. The following chart shows a summary and comparison of all three sources of information.

The order in which the waganga placed the frequency of the types of cases coming to them is summarized in the chart under columns A, B and C. Column A lists the total number of times the type of problem was listed by the waganga as being one of the problems brought to them. Sickness and sorcery were each listed sixty times by the sixty waganga.

TABLE 3: Summary of Waganga and Client Case Studies

Category of problem brought to the waganga	No. of times given position	The order in which the waganga placed the frequency of cases they treated	The order of frequency according to the waganga	No. of cases treated by waganga on previous day	Problems of 100 Zaramo brought to waganga in Dar es Salaam
SICKNESS	60	57 gave 1st place 3 gave 2nd place	1st	338	12 (51 additional cases listed under other categories) Total 63
SORCERY	60	36 gave 1st place 21 gave 2nd place 3 gave 3rd place	2nd	158	43 (20 additional sorcery cases under other categories) Total 63 43 of these sickness
PROTECTION	57	29 gave 1st place 25 gave 2nd place 3 gave 3rd place	3rd	120	5
WORK	46	2 gave 1st place 3 gave 2nd place 10 gave 3rd place 16 gave 4th place 10 gave 5th place 5 gave 6th place	4th	11	5
SEXUAL PROBLEMS	37	2 gave 1st place 1 gave 2nd place 10 gave 3rd place 11 gave 4th place 10 gave 5th place 3 gave 6th place	5th	2	1
BUSINESS PROBLEMS	29	1 gave 1st place 4 gave 2nd place 6 gave 3rd place 10 gave 4th place 7 gave 5th place 1 gave 6th place	6th	2	3 (all involved sorcery)
SPIRITS & RITUAL OBLIGATIONS	22	1 gave 3rd place 6 gave 4th place 9 gave 5th place 6 gave 6th place	7th	2	10 (7 of these involved sickness)

TABLE 3: Cont.

Category of problem brought to the waganga	No. of times given position	The order in which the waganga placed the frequency of cases they treated	The order of frequency according to the waganga	No. of cases treated by waganga on previous day	Problems of 100 Zaramo brought to waganga in Dar es Salaam
MARITAL PROBLEMS	11	3 gave 4th place 4 gave 5th place 4 gave 6th place	8th	-	7 (6 of these involved sorcery)
SPORTS	6	1 gave3rd place 1 gave 4th place 1 gave 5th place 3 gave 6th place	9th	-	-
POLITICS	2	2 gave 5th place	10th	-	-
MENTAL ILLNESS	-	some said only a few cases each month	-	3	7
COURT AND PRISON CASES AND THEFT	-	some said only a few cases each month	-	-	4 court *3 theft* 7 total
MISCEL-LANEOUS	-	some said a few 'good luck' cases each month	-	-	-
TOTAL				636 cases (from 60 waganga)	

With this overall summary of the frequency and placement of the Zaramo's urban problems we shall now return to each category separately to examine the cases and problems in detail.

1. Sickness

If any people in Dar es Salaam become physically sick, *mgonjwa*, Sw., it is possible for them to receive medication in a dispensary or hospital free of charge. It is understandable that a person whose illness is thought to be caused by a spirit, a neglected rite or sorcery might wish to go to a traditional medicine man, but it is less understandable why a person should seek his aid for normal illness, paying a considerable price for the treatment when free treatment could be obtained at a clinic.

At the time this investigation was made there were in Dar es Salaam one major 600-bed hospital, one maternity clinic, one private hospital, nine government clinics and one Roman Catholic clinic. In addition to this there were no fewer than 20 private doctors located mainly in the center of the city. A number of larger factories also had medical services for their workers, of whom the majority are men. The traditional medicine men are located in the residential areas where most of the non-European and Asian population live.

One obvious reason then for Zaramo to go to traditional medicine men is that they are within easy reach. With very few private cars available, patients must ride crowded buses and walk long distances to get to the hospital, so it is easier to visit a mganga living in the neighborhood. An even more understandable reason for avoiding Government clinics or hospitals might be the crowded conditions, the long waiting lines and the cursory treatment given by overworked doctors and nurses.

A few facts reported by Dr. A.D. Chiduo, the Medical Superintendent of the Dar es Salaam Group of Hospitals, give evidence of the overcrowded conditions.[1]

> ". . . The truth is that doctors are being very much overworked. To just quote an example, take Mnazi Moja dispensary. This has only seven doctors inclusive of medical assistants and in one single month - in January, they handled 192,928 patients and this actually meant attending about 326 patients every day. It means that each doctor or medical assistant working non-stop for 24 hours could give each patient five minutes. . . Muhimbili (hospital) has 31 registered medical officers for 1,200 beds . . . plus 200-250 patients daily on the floor while Mulengo Hospital in Kampala has 90 registered medical officers for 1,160 beds. Muhimbili Hospital has an additional 12 medical specialists on the staff compared with 44 specialists in Mulengo Hospital in Kampala."

This information illustrates the difficult situation for both doctors and patients alike and shows why people might prefer to go to a traditional mganga. One reason suggested as to why the government may not wish to officially forbid the work of the traditional waganga is that the official health services can hardly cope with all the cases which already come to them. To forbid the waganga to practise would only add additional thousands of patients to the already overloaded system.

Six of the twelve clients being treated by waganga for sickness had first gone to the hospital, dispensary or private doctor before going to the medicine man. Of the remaining 88 clients out of the 100, an additional 12 (13.6 per cent) had gone first to a hospital or clinic before going to the waganga.

Among the twelve cases being treated for sickness, the six who had first visited a hospital, dispensary or doctor said that they had decided to try a local mganga because they were not cured. In some cases it appears that they left the hospital treatment far too early for it to have had a curative effect on their illness. In three of the six cases the first mganga was also unsuccessful with his treatment and the client had left to try another mganga. If the stomach trouble, *chango*, happened to be an ulcer or tumor, or any number of other problems, no medicine, whoever dispensed it, would cure the person in a matter of days or even a few weeks. Unfortunately, it is a rather common practice to switch from dispensary to hospital care, or from mganga to mganga, if there is no quick relief.

One patient, the only male amongst the twelve sickness cases, had tuberculosis and had previously spent six months in a hospital. He had been released several months before, but the symptoms returned. Since he did not wish to go to the hospital again, he sent his brother to a mganga in Burguruni to get medicine. The mganga gave the brother several blue papers with portions of the Koran written on it. He was told to put the papers into a white bottle and fill it with water. The sick man was to drink this blue water twice a day. A week later the brother was interviewed again and he said that the patient's condition was not good and he thought the medicine he had received from the mganga was not good. He stated: "I don't think that written words could turn into medicine and cure my brother." He decided to take his brother back to his home in the country near Maneromango, where he believed he would get "proper medicine" from the waganga there. After some weeks of treatment in the country the brother began to spit blood and they finally agreed to take him to the government hospital.

In six cases the client had not gone to a hospital/dispensary but went directly to a local mganga. Four of these spoke of "my mganga" as one to whom they always turned and who had previously been successful in treating their problems. One client considered all medicines alike and, as she was helped by local medicine, saw no need to get to a hospital for treatment.

The husband of one patient would not send his wife to the hospital for her stomach trouble because he thought the doctors there played with his wife's sexual organs. In earlier times there was a reluctance on the part of women to be examined by male doctors, but this does not appear to be the case today. As there is no physical examination whatsoever with the traditional waganga, it may be that women who are shy or object to being examined by a doctor prefer to go to a local mganga.

Nine of the twelve cases of sickness were called *chango*, Sw., stomach trouble. *Chango* is the general term given to any ailment in the abdominal area, and it is also the name for the small intestines as well as the name for round intestinal worms. *Chango* problems could be caused by worms or stomach ulcers, as often seems to be case, but it could be a kidney, liver or other problem. The waganga seem to ask no detailed questions of the clients about their *chango* ailments. The medicine given is supposed to cure whatever is wrong, be it worms, ulcers or tumors.

Four of the twelve cases had been diagnosed by a diviner. The eight others understood their case to be illness only, without the help of a diviner. When diviners are allowed to diagnose the cases, as we shall see later in the other categories, a greater percentage of the sickness problems are attributed to sorcery. Out of the 43 sorcery cases, 38 had physical illnesses which were treated by the waganga. Seven of the 10 spirit cases were treated for physical illness, and five of the seven marital cases included physical illness. Out of the 100 cases, a total of 63 were treated for physical illness, but the diagnosis of the diviner credited the illness to the work of sorcery and not to biological or natural causes.

It is evident from the prevalence of sickness cases brought to the waganga that the greatest single role of waganga in Zaramo society is still that of healer. Regardless of the reasons given for the cause of the illness and regardless of his additional functions, the mganga's major activity is the practice of medicine for the purpose of bodily therapy. Even if a growing number of Zaramo go to hospital for treatment, the mganga is considered a successful medical practitioner in the eyes of the local people. As a medicine man his reputation is good and his clients not only return to him but recommend him to the others. Thus the role of the mganga as a physical healer continues side by side with "Western, scientific" medical practitioners. If 338 sickness cases treated in a single day by 60 waganga can be considered average, there must be between 3,000 and 4,000 people treated for illness by waganga each day throughout the city. This no doubt equals in number the people attending Government medical facilities and well confirms the mganga's role as a healer in Zaramo society.

2. Sorcery

In order to describe the accusations of sorcery found in Dar es Salaam, I am providing the reader with a brief summary of the 43 sorcery cases revealed in the 100 cases treated by waganga in the city.

These 43 cases will show the range of this problem in Zaramo society and the relationship between the accused and the accuser. The participation of the mganga/diviner who builds up the fear of sorcery and confirms the activity of the *mchawi* through his divination revelations should be noted. Although the majority of the victims of sorcery experience bodily and mental illness, it may be seen in Table 4 why they did not take their case to the government hospital. Following the summaries found in the Table, other additional information will be given as well as the analysis.

The medicine men in Dar es Salaam listed sorcery as the number two problem which people bring to them. As stated previously, dealing with sorcery may mean curing the individual of illness or of the misfortune caused by the sorcerer. It may include ridding clients of the sorcerer's poison or power in their bodies as well as protecting them from further intrusions. Like-wise, it may include revenge or punishment to the accused evildoer. This revenge may be in the form of a curse, of magical sympathetic rites, or of actual poison and other actions intended to harm the accused person.

I have tried to group these cases into various categories for analysis, but some of them are so complex they could be included under a number of different problem headings. Table 4 gives a break down of 43 general sorcery cases. Discussion of these will be followed by a description of mental cases, marital cases, business problems and protection cases, all involving sorcery or the fear of it.

TABLE 4: Sorcery Treated by Waganga

DATA FROM 43 CASES IN DAR ES SALAAM

Case No.	Sex	Diviner used?	Symptom of problem	Cause	Relationship to accused	Did client first go to government hospital for treatment? Comments.
1 S.1[2]	F	Yes	Whole body sick; about to die.	Sorcery - a *jini*. Jealous of my child. She hasn't any.	Neighbor in same house. Female	No. We knew it was a *jini* so there was no need to go to a hospital.
2 S.5	F	Yes	Coughing	Sorcery - hatred of a witch (Mwanga)	Female neighbor.	No. Went to have a *halubadili* read. If she tries it again she will die.
3 S.6	F	Yes	Heart trouble	Sorcery - poison. Jealous of my salary.	Female neighbor.	Yes. Went many months to government hospital. Did not get proper *dawa*.
4 S.7	F	Yes	*Uchawi* put at room door.	Sorcery - hatred of neighbor.	Female neighbor.	No. Was sent to an mganga by a friend.
5 S.9	F	Yes	*Chembe cha moyo* - pain in the heart.	Sorcery - female neighbor wrongly suspects me with her husband	Female neighbor, same house.	Yes. Went to dispensary for 5 days; was not helped. Diviner told me I was bewitched by neighbour.
6 S.10	F	Yes	Pregnancy almost a year old.	Sorcery. She did this because of quarrel.	Female neighbor.	No. Because this was *uchawi* sorcery, i did not think it necessary to go to pre-natal clinic or hospital.
7 S.12	F	Yes	Stomach trouble - *chango*	Sorcery. The mganga said there is a woman who hates me.	Female neighbor.	No. Went first to a diviner. Then to the mganga.
8 S.13	F	Yes	Chest aches	Sorcery - poison.	Female neighbor in same house.	No hospital treatment.
9 S.16	M	Yes	*Kipanda uso* - headache on forehead.	Sorcery - African poison. Revenge by woman I chased.	Woman friend	Yes. Went to private doctor for one week. Was not successful because it was *sumu ya kiswahili* African (Swahili) poison.
10 S.18	F	Yes	Stomach trouble. There is a thing in the stomach.	Sorcery - My father has a house. A cousin wants to kill me to get it.	Cousin, male	Yes. Went to private doctor for two weeks. An African poison cannot be treated in a hospital.

TABLE 4: Cont.

Case No.	Sex	Diviner used?	Symptom of problem	Cause	Relationship to accused	Did client first go to government hospital for treatment? Comments.
11 S.18	M	Yes	Whole body was sick.	Sorcery - a *jini* was put to kill me for revenge.	Neighbours living in village where man is magistrate. Revenge for his court case verdicts	Went to hospital only one day. His wife and a diviner convinced him it was sorcery so he took the mganga treatment.
12 S.20	M	Yes	Leg aching	Sorcery - stepped on *uchawi* poison by mistake. It was not meant for me.	Not known. Accidental.	Yes. Went 3 days to clinic. *Uchawi* cannot be treated by European medicine.
13 S.21	F	No	*Kichomi* ache on side.	Sorcery - hatred, *sumu ya kiswahili* - poison of Swahili people.	Realtive - in same Zaramo clan.	No hospital treatment. My husband sent me here. He knew this mganga.
14 S.22	F	Yes	Legs ache.	Sorcery - stepped on *uchawi* which was not meant for me.	Not known. Accidental.	Yes. Went 3 days to clinic. *Uchawi* cannot be treated by European medicine.
15 S.29	F	Yes	*Hizi* - menstrual bleeding doesn't stop.	Sorcery - stepped on trap of *dawa* Wife suspects me of going out with her husband.	Female neighbor in same house. Another tribe (Ngoni).	Yes. Dispensary treatment for 3 days was not successful.
16 S.32	M	Yes	Has bad dreams - carving dead bodies, dancing naked.	Sorcery - it is the work of a witch.	Suspects old woman (witch) living in next room.	No. I did not go to a hospital because I knew it was a witch trying to harm me.
17 S.33	M	Yes	*Kichomi* - ache on side.	Sorcery - neighbour is jealous of my good business. He wants to pull me down so that I leave the business.	Male neighbour of another tribe (Rufiji). Also a fruit and vegetable seller.	No hospital treatment.

TABLE 4: Cont.

Case No.	Sex	Diviner used?	Symptom of problem	Cause	Relationship to accused	Did client first go to government hospital for treatment? Comments.
18 S.34	F	Yes	Stomach troubles.	Sorcery - Mganga said neighbor is jealous of my clothing and food. Must move away before she kills me.	Female, old woman is accused. There was no trouble before divining was made.	Yes. Went to private doctors first but in vain.
19 S.36	F	Yes	Stomach troubles.	Sorcery - I was bewitched.	Female - (would not tell more).	Yes. Went to the hospital for a long time. Works there. Also tried other waganga without good results.
20 S.37	M	No	Fever and bad dreams. Body aches all over.	Sorcery - witches use him at nights to carry dead corpses.	Witch not known.	No hospital treatment. Went to mganga to buy amulet protection against witches.
21 S.42	F	No	Had bad dream. Woke up spitting blood and coughing.	Sorcery - I was bewitched.	Female neighbors. Two women hate her,	No hospital treatment. Went to a *shehe*
22 S.53	F	?	?	Sorcery	Female neighbor living in same house.	No hospital treatment. "They knew it was *uchawi* and it can't be treated in a hospital."
23 S.54	F	?	Fever - She stepped on a large dead lizard in her room.	Sorcery - The *mchawi* dropped this dead lizard in her room.	Not known yet.	No hospital treatment. Has gone to several other waganga but is still sick.
24 S.55	F	Yes	Bad dream - eating human flesh; vomited; has since had pain in stomach	Sorcery - according to mganga a witch did it to me.	Witch, female living next house.	No hospital treatment. "Quite sure clinics can't treat this." Now with second maganga.
25 S.59	M	Yes	Bit by a snake in an open place.	Sorcery - it was sent by someone to kill.	Not known yet.	No hospital treatment. I knew it was *uchawi* sent by someone.

TABLE 4: Cont.

Case No.	Sex	Diviner used?	Symptom of problem	Cause	Relationship to accused	Did client first go to government hospital for treatment? Comments.
26 S.60	M	Yes	"Very sick"	I was told it was sorcery by mganga / diviner.	Diviner said I was bewitched by my mother, but she had died 5 years previously.	First went to diviner. After he told patient it was his mother he did not believe it. Now going second month to hospital.
27 S.63	F	Yes	"Very sick"	Sorcery - neighbous hate and are jealous of my large *shamba*, garden.	Neighbors living in same village. Man who bewitched her died of revenge	No hospital treatment. She was brought by her son to the city for treatment, protection and revenge*dawa* for herself and her*shamba.*
28 S.64	M	?	School boy does poorly at school. A *dudu*, bug creature, runs inside his body.	Sorcery - another boy who did not get into school is jealous.	Neighbour boy.	No hospital treatment. His father took him to a mganga.
29 S.65	M Boy	Yes	2 yr. old child vomits, *chango.*	Sorcery - *Hemas* herb poison and menstrual blood mixed in food.	Female neighbor who does not have child is jealous of her baby.	No hospital treatment. The diviner sent her to present mganga for *dawa.*
30 S.66	F	Yes	Sick. Something was thrown at her and her child.	Sorcery - Wife of owner of house is jealous of her child. She wants to kill both.	Female neighbor living in same house. Uses bad language to this woman.	Yes. Went to dispensary for one week. Suspected sorcery so went to a diviner and was told this.
31 S.68	F	Yes	*Kihanda uso* - forehead aches.	Sorcery-diviner told her it was *uchawi.*	Could not say.	No hospital treatment. *Uchawi* cannot be treated in hospitals.
32 S.69	F	Yes	Pregnancy 10 months old.	Sorcery-diviner said she was bewitched.	Would not say.	No hospital treatment. Because diviner said she was bewitched; "Clinics therefore cannot help."
33 S.70	M	Yes	*Chembe cha moyo* - heart trouble.	Sorcery - hatred and revenge by cousin who thinks his mother killed his father.	Mother's brother's son with whom he has quarrelled over a sorcery accusation.	No hospital treatment. "I know it is sorcery and the diviner has also said it is sorcery."

TABLE 4: Cont.

Case No.	Sex	Diviner used?	Symptom of problem	Cause	Relationship to accused	Did client first go to government hospital for treatment? Comments.
34 S.71	F	?	Stomach trouble - swelling.	Sorcery - was given meat to eat by neighbor, got sick after it.	Female neighbor who lives in same house.	Yes. Went to hospital but they failed to help her so had to go to mganga. (She works in a hospital.)
35 S.74	M	Yes	Seriously sick. About to die.	Sorcery - A man caught me in adultery with his wife: did this for revenge.	Male neighbour.	No hospital treatment. "They all know..." and the diviner also said he was bewitched by another husband.
36 S.75	F	?	Stomach trouble.	Sorcery	Female neighbor living in same house.	No hospital treatment. Husband sent for village mganga to treat his wife.
37 S.76	F	?	Sick	Sorcery - female houseowner hated me very much. There was no reason.	Female house-owner living in same house.	No hospital treatment. After treatment by mganga she moved to a different house.
38 S.77	F	Yes	Sick	Sorcery - neighbor jealous of my good food and clothes.	Female neighbor in same house.	No hospital treatment. Mganga called in from home village. Treatment given at crossroads.
39 S.78	M	Yes	Sick	Sorcery - co-worker wrongly suspects me of having relations with his wife.	A male co-worker (prison warder). A diviner said he had bewitched him for revenge.	Yes. Was in two different hospitals for several weeks each. But it was only local medicines which cured me.
40 S.80	M	Yes	Cats were crying at the window at night. Sometimes hyenas came	Sorcery - he believes his father's mother in whose house he lives is a *mchawi* and wants to bewitch him as well as his parents.	His father's mother. She owns the house where he is living with his parents. Father went for *ramli* and told him this.	No hospital treatment. The boy moved from the house. Now only comes to greet his father and mother but does not stay. (His father perhaps wanted the boy to move out of the house, using sorcery as an excuse.)
41 S.81	M	No	Sick in bed for several months. Fear of being killed.	Forced to cut up a dead body which would be used for sorcery purposes. Became sick after this.	Prostitute female friend and several of her accomplices. Forced him by threat.	No hospital treatment. Relatives brought mganga for treatment. They knew what the cause was. (This might have been a dream, but told as an actual event in Dar.)

TABLE 4: Cont.

Case No.	Sex	Diviner used?	Symptom of problem	Cause	Relationship to accused	Did client first go to government hospital for treatment? Comments.
42 S.83	S	Yes	Menstrual bleeding did not stop.	Sorcery - neighbor hates me. I do not know why.	Female neighbor in same house. She thinks she may have inherited her *uchawi.*	Yes. Went to hospital first but wasn't helped. A diviner then told her what her trouble was and who did it. (*Mzimu* and *dawa* treatment.)
43 S.84	F	?	Very sick. (70-80 years old)	Sorcery - neighbors jealous and hate her. Tried to kill her because of good fortune. Clothes, money and helpful children.	Her neighbours bewitched and killed her husband. Now they try to kill her.	No hospital treatment. "She could not be helped in a hospital. Only a local mganga can help *uchawi* ."

The following patterns should be noted: 38 clients were female; 24 were male; one case was a husband and wife seeking treatment together: total 63. This means that approximately 60 per cent of the cases were women, and 38 per cent men. Out of the total of 100 cases 54 involved women, 40 involved men, 3 included a husband and wife together and 3 concerned babies or small children. Within the total group therefore there is a slightly higher percentage of women than men troubled with problems of sorcery.

These figures indicate that women may be less adjusted to urban life than men. Generally living in one room, crowded with other families in the same house, sharing cooking and toilet facilities in the courtyard, women have more opportunity than men to become irritated with their neighbors. Petty remarks and suspicions between these women often develop into accusations of sorcery. Men on the other hand have a daily change from their living quarters when they go off to work. They have friends at work, they visit bars, go to football games and often spend evenings visiting friends in other parts of town. Women are generally confined to their small living area. For this reason women have more opportunity for frustrations which give rise to the higher percentage involved in sorcery accusations.

The case studies reveal that the majority of sorcery accusations by women were levelled at female neighbors living in the same house. Out of the 43 sorcery accusations only two female accusations were against males - in one case against a male cousin, and the other a man in a home village.

The 24 accusations by bewitched males were levelled at 10 males, 6 females and 8 unknown people. Of the 10 accusations against males, 3 were against co-workers and 3 against competitors in business, again people with whom there was a close social contact. The cases against females involved sexual and marital tensions. From the urban sorcery cases in Dar es Salaam we can conclude that most accusations are made against people with whom there is close social intercourse. Tensions evidenced in the cases are not due to social, economic, educational or religious stratification, nor to competition for power or authority. It is seen in the cases that the accused and the accusers are generally people on the same social level.

Of the total 63 sorcery cases, only 4 were accusations against members of the same kin group. Even one of these happened to be a jealous co-worker in the same hospital. In this, the urban situation in Dar es Salaam differs from many of the rural situations where the tensions and accusations are mainly between kin group members.

The evidence from my cases would fully support Max Marwick (1970, 17) when he states: "The relative frequency of accusations in various social relationships provides us with a set of social strain-gauges for detecting where the tensions and role-conflicts in a particular society lie." Whereas in his Cewa society study the predominant conflict area was within the matrilineage, in this urban study the conflict and tensions arise between neighbors who are in daily contact or with co-workers with whom there is competition for jobs. The other urban social strain area shown in the case material is in marriage and love affairs. Because close kin support and tribal sanctions are lacking in the city, in many situations couples in conflict resort to sorcery as a way of dealing with their marital problems. All male sorcery accusations against women involved martial problems or love affairs.

Marc Swartz (1969, 25-33) rightly states that most students of witchcraft and sorcery in Africa agree in believing that witchcraft accusations are a reflection of interpersonal tensions. He summarizes Marwick's view that witchcraft accusations will occur when there is tension between individuals due to their competition for some highly valued end; second, that these same individuals are united in co-operation in other contexts; and third, that their roles in the competition are not clearly defined and delimited.

Both Swartz and Marwick (1970, 379-382) then pose the question: If the above hypothesis is correct, then shouldn't the urban "modernization" processes which cause social strain because of employment and position competition, martial and sexual relationships, business competition, and inter-tribal relationships result in the increase of witchcraft accusations in urban society. If the sources of interpersonal conflict which lead to witch craft accusations have increased in the cities, then on theoretical grounds the frequency of witchcraft accusations should be on the increase. Mitchell (1965) and Swartz (1969), however, came to the opposite conclusion. On both assertions my material casts objections.

Swartz, for example, states: ". . . although witchcraft accusations and belief have increased in rural areas there is some fairly persuasive evidence to indicate that in urban areas there is less witchcraft accusation and, perhaps, less witchcraft - based explanation of misfortune than there is in the rural areas." Swartz admits that he has no empirical data to measure the increase or decrease of urban accusations. He discounts the use of court cases as reliable evidence, noting that very few cases are brought to the courts in cities and that the laws which oppose witchcraft accusations would deter anyone from making such an official accusation in the first place. Swartz concludes "tentatively" that there is less witchcraft accusation among townsmen than among villagers, on the basis of Bena informants who had lived in cities but who were back in their villages when contacted. He does not state the number interviewed or in which cities or towns these Bena lived.

I agree with Swartz that an anthropologist living amongst the Bena may receive a fuller picture of the actual situation than court records or statistics could reveal, but I would be very cautions about making generalizations from what I know about the Bena or Zaramo, or any one ethnic group, asserting that they are typical of all ethnic groups living in urban areas. A strong traditional religious group and a Muslim community may differ considerably from each other in beliefs and practise as regards witchcraft and sorcery. The Bena are not typical of Tanzania's population, urban or rural, hence a wide sample would have to be made to get any conclusive pattern.

Information received retrospectively does not give as reliable evidence as that gained on the spot.

According to my survey, about 5,000 cases every day in Dar es Salaam concerned accusations of witchcraft and sorcery. This cannot be considered an insignificant number. It indicates a very troublesome area in urban society. It was noted earlier that the actual number of medicine men in the city compares favorably with the rural village area of Bunju. We do not know what the figures for practising medicine men or for witchcraft accusations were 20 or 50 years ago, so we cannot at this time determine whether there is an increase or decline. It may be possible ten years hence to make a study in the same areas to determine the trend. Even if the ratio of practising waganga in the rural and urban areas is the same, it is evident that the case load of Dar es Salaam urban medicine men is much greater. It is a full-time business, whereas in Bunju it was practised together with agriculture and fishing.

The argument that Mitchell (1965, 202) puts forth for "the decline of witchcraft accusations in urban areas" is that the social and administrative structure of the urban community allows a person no direct retributive action. There is a tendency to see misfortune ultimately then in terms of the action of the angered spirits of a deceased kinsman. My Dar es Salaam material and the Bunju rural case material contradicts this completely. While it is true that the Zaramo can no longer take the suspected sorcerer to court, nor is one allowed to burn a witch as in olden days, the supposed victims still have possibilities for effective retributive action which apparently satisfies them. They can firstly be treated with the medicine to take away the evil spell or power; they can get protective medicine so that it will not recur, and finally they can read a curse against the suspected evildoers or may take secret revenge by using their own acquired magical power or poison. All of this may indeed be magical action against unknown or mystical suspects, but the accusers are satisfied that they took "effective action." Or, as many cases reveal, the "effective action" was simply to move to another part of the city to avoid confrontation.

Mitchell's theory that urban dwellers avoid making witchcraft accusations by seeing their misfortune in terms of angered spirits is further contradicted by the urban-rural data used in this research. In the rural Bunju study, out of a total of 62 cases treated by a rural medicine man, 36 (58 per cent) were said to be calamities caused by spirit intervention, while the smaller number, 17 (27.5 per cent), were ascribed to sorcery. The opposite was found to be true in Dar es Salaam. Out of 100 cases treated by urban waganga, only 10 (10 per cent) were said to be caused by spirits and 63 per cent were ascribed to sorcery. Because the urban medicine man and his client find it difficult to treat or exorcise a troubling spirit in the city, they tend to diagnose the cause as sorcery, which they can handle. This exactly proves Mitchell's other contention that "Town Africans in the main continue to interpret their misfortune in 'personal' terms but the final meaning they attach to the misfortune must be of a type which will allow them to take effective action" (1965, 201). In this case "effective action" is easier to take against sorcery than against a spirit.

Swartz and Mitchell fail to note sufficiently in their analysis the operative difference between a witch and a sorcerer. Mitchell's cases seem to refer to accusations against witches. Swartz lumps the work of witches and sorcerers together, calling it 'witchcraft' (1969, 25). The evidence is much clearer if we make a distinction between accusations against witches and accusations against people who use methods of sorcery for evil intent. If Mitchell means that there are fewer accusations against witches in urban areas I belive he is correct. But there are not fewer accusations against those practising sorcery. It seems that in the minds of most Central Africans witches and sorcerers are one and the same person, whereas in Coastal Tanzania there is a fine distinction. A witch, to a Zaramo, is a person who has power which is inherent in the witch's person, while a sorcerer must rely on medicine, spells, ceremony and magical acts and objects. Whereas the witch acts according to his or her nature and does so mainly for self-gratification, a sorcerer is generally employed by others to do the deeds of evil. Urban Zaramo informants all believed in the reality of witches and believed that some do still exist, but they claimed that there are fewer of them these days in the city. On the other hand, sorcery is on the increase. Because of the urban competition and tensions, people have more reason to believe that a co-worker or neighbor has evil intent and has applied some form of magic or poison against them. They do not believe that the neighbor or co-worker flies through the night, changes into an owl or hyena or dances naked in the moonlight, as is the common assumption about witches. Swartz argues that the processes of "modernization" and the "major proselytizing religions" have substantially eradicated or seriously weakened beliefs in supernatural agencies (1969, 26). While this seems to be true for belief in the activity of witches, it has not weakened belief in sorcery activity not performed by witches.

From the case material we might ask whether the plots of sorcery were real or just imagined by the accuser? Did the neighbor actually poison the client, as was claimed in Cases 3, 9, 12, 13 and 29? Were all the other sicknesses listed the result of a sorcerer's power and were they actually instigated by a neighbor? The evidence shows that the majority of these accusations were either suggested or confirmed by the diviner. He was careful, as was his client, not to accuse a particular person by name, for which he could be taken to court. Instead, the diviner, knowing the general tensions in urban society, suggested a neighbor as the culprit, knowing the client would have one or two people in mind on whom blame could be pinned.

The persons designated as witches or sorcerers in these cases may have been entirely innocent of the actions attributed to them, but the faulty relationship between the accuser and the accused was undoubtedly very real. In the majority of cases listed, the accuser gave either hatred or jealousy as the reason for the misdeed. The real jealousy and hatred might, however, be the reverse of what was stated. It may well be the projection of the accuser's animosity against the accused. The young boy in Case 40 knew that he was not wanted in the house of his father's mother. There was little he could do to change the situation. Therefore it may have given him some consolation to think that his father's mother was a witch and that he had better leave the house. A male worker, Case S. 23, was no doubt having difficulty in keeping his job, due to psychopathic disorder. Rather than accepting or understanding his own incapabilities, it was convenient to project his fear or inner tension by accusing a co-worker of bewitching him.

An additional factor often giving rise to accusations of sorcery is the failure of hospital treatment or that given by a private doctor. One third of the sorcery case clients had first gone to a hospital or clinic. After a few days or a week, when they saw no results, they left to seek help from a traditional mganga. In most cases they left too early, not giving the medication time to take effect. Because traditionalists believe "Western medicine" cannot cure sorcery, they jump to the conclusion that, as they are not getting better immediately, their problem must be due to sorcery. If the diviner knows that the client coming to him has first gone to a hospital and has not been successfully cured, he knows that his diagnosis of sorcery will be readily accepted.

The manner in which sorcery was experienced by the clients often involved sickness. In several cases bad dreams accompanied sickness. Table 5 gives a summary.

TABLE 5: Symptoms of Sorcery

The Manner in Which Sorcery Was Experienced by 63 Zaramo of Dar es Salaam

Symptoms	*Number*
Physical sickness (stomach pains, heart palpitations, coughing, general body aches)	40
Mental illness (depression)	6
Intense fear (of death, sickness or about property)	6
Bad dreams	4
Object thrown or placed in house of victim	4
Business failing	3
Abnormal menstruation period	2
Abnormal pregnancy period	2
Snake bite	1
Unknown	1

Almost two-thirds of all sorcery clients attributed their physical illness to the work of sorcery. Because of their lack of scientific understanding as to the nature and cause of illness, they were ready to believe that the physical illness was willed by someone or inflicted on them with poison or through an object. Who? Why? How? were the questions troubling the client, and which were presented to the medicine man.

Most of the bodily problems were not unusual, but followed very much the same pattern as the problems of those who thought their sickness was due to natural causes. Stomach trouble, *chango*, was found to be the most common problem, although the specific stomach ailment was not known. Heart pains, headaches, fever and aches of all kinds were likewise attributed to the work of sorcery.

These ailments were believed to have entered the body by means of poison, *sumu ya kiswahili*, Sw., placed in food or sent through the air in some mysterious manner. In some cases a *jini* was thought to have entered the body. In several cases a client claimed to have stepped on *uchawi* poison or a "thing", but this poison or thing, like the *jini*, was never visible. In the majority of cases the clients could not specify the means by which the sorcery came upon them. It was assumed to be by some mysterious, magical means conducted by a professional sorcerer at the request of an enemy who had paid for it.

Sorcery was also thought to be the cause in the cases of two abnormally long pregnancies. The first woman said that her pregnancy was almost one year old. She had not gone to a pre-natal clinic and was not willing to do so because she firmly believed "the problem is *uchawi*." The diviner had revealed her problem was the work of sorcery and since she had once quarreled with a neighbor she believed it was this person who had now bewitched her. She went to this same mganga for medicine and felt that the baby would now come. The second woman, who already had two children, claimed that she was ten months pregnant at the time of the interview. She was naturally worried and had gone to a diviner to learn the source of her problem. The diviner told her she had been bewitched and unless she went to a mganga for medicine she would not be able to give birth to her baby. The woman began taking medicine from a mganga and rejected advice that she visit a Government doctor. She said she had been bewitched and that she could not be helped in a clinic.

It is difficult to asses the pregnancy problem of these two women and to know whether or not they were overdue or if they had simply miscalculated their dates. It is common belief among the Zaramo that a *mchawi* has the power to "dry up" or take an unborn baby from a pregnant woman. For this reason the Zaramo women traditionally secluded themselves and avoided public gatherings during the time of pregnancy, for fear that someone would take or kill their unborn child. Because witches and *wachawi* claim such powers, and because the waganga and diviners give credit to this claim by offering cures and protection for pregnant women, the belief still persists. The waganga are the chief agents in perpetuating this *uchawi* belief because they confirm the fears traditionally harbored by the Zaramo.

In this present day we could say the mganga has assumed the role of an obstetrician but, rather than dealing with the real pregnancy, he ascribes the difficulty to sorcery. The result could be disastrous for the women and babies.

a. *Witches*:
In 5 cases the *mchawi*, sorcerer, was specified as a witch, *mwanga*, Sw. All five witches were said to be female, two being specified as "old women." One accuser, a boy, agreed with his father and the diviner's verdict that the witch was his father's mother who was trying to get rid of him. Among these five cases, three of the accusers were male and two were female.

Bad dreams in many parts of Africa are associated with the work of witches, and so also amongst the Zaramo. Client S.32 claimed he had dreams in which he found himself carving up dead bodies and dancing naked. He did not need a diviner to tell him the cause of such dreams, nor was it necessary for him to go to a hospital; it was obvious to him that a witch was using him to do her evil work at night. He suspected the witch to be an old woman living in the room next to his.

Client S.37, a male, also had bad dreams from which he awoke with fever and bodily aches. He said witches were using him to carry corpses at night, hence his body ached from tiredness in the morning. He also did not need the elucidation of a diviner, but went directly to a mganga to buy an amulet for protection. He did not know who the witch was.

Client S.55 repeatedly dreamt that she was eating human flesh. She awakened with pains in her stomach and vomited. According to her diviner/mganga, the problem was induced by a witch. The client added, "I am quite sure hospital clinics can't treat this." She suspected a female neighbor living in the same house to be the witch. Because eating flesh, dancing naked and carrying dead bodies in dreams are always associated with the work of witches, these clients readily assumed their dreams were also the work of witches.

Client S.5 had a female neighbor who, she said, hated her and therefore caused her coughing fits. She referred to this neighbor as a *mwanga*, witch, but I doubt if she believed her to be a witch who flies in the night and can change herself into an animal. Possibly she called her neighbor a "witch" only in a derogatory sense. She went to a Muslim practitioner to have a *halubadili* read so that, "If she tries again she will die."

Client S.80 (Case 40) was a boy about 16 years old who lived with his parents in the house of his father's mother. At night he imagined he heard cats crying at his window and sometimes hyenas. When the father went to a diviner for *ramli* he was told that the boy's paternal grandmother was a witch and was intending to bewitch the boy as well as the parents. The boy subsequently moved away from the house, but the parents remained there. It seems apparent that because of crowded conditions which made it necessary for the boy to share the same room with his parents, the father may have used the boy's problem as an excuse to move him out. In this case I am doubtful if the father actually went to a diviner for *ramli* but may have made up the story to convince his son that he should quickly leave the house.

In these five cases the clients dealt with their witch problems in various ways, the complete treatment not always being revealed. The boy moved away; another client bought a protective amulet; one woman had a *halubadili* read; the others may have used medicine for their stomach pains and fever as well as taking "appropriate" protective measures.

b. *Mental Illness*:

Mental illness in Zaramo society is viewed as an indisputable sign of sorcery. This is the case also in other African societies. T. Adeoye Lambo's study of a group of mentally ill Nigerian students in Great Britain revealed that 90 per cent of the patients believed their problem to be that of bewitchment and the machinations of an enemy (1964, 445).

Six of the seven mental cases found amongst the 100 interviewed cases credited their malady to *uchawi*. The one mentally ill client who did not think the cause to be sorcery was an adolescent Christian school-girl. All other six mental patients were Muslims.

Among these seven cases, four were female and three were male clients. Three had gone to a hospital for treatment but, like the others, had no confidence in modern cures. One, while in the hospital, was receiving traditional medicine brought in by his relatives. The other two commented: "They couldn't help me at the hospital because I was bewitched." Another client went to the hospital because it was the only way to claim sick leave pay from his employer. Others who had not bothered to go to the Government hospital typically commented: "The Government can't help this; they can't cure *uchawi*; we knew it was *uchawi* from the beginning, so we came here."

Four of the seven mental cases had gone to a diviner to find out who had made them mentally ill. In two cases I did not receive the diviner's verdict and only in the case of the Christian girl was it specifically stated that a diviner had not been consulted.

Here we have reason to question the diviner's diagnosis of the problem. He may know good techniques in handling his client, but does he do society justice by suggesting that all mental illness is due to sorcery? He may relieve the client's neurosis, but the social damage done between neighbors, co-workers and family members may be even more tragic than the original neurotic state of the client.

Because traditional believers with mental illness have little trust in Western medicine, Nigerian psychiatrist Lambo has tried to combine indigenous psychotherapeutic practices with his own hospital services. Mental patients were encouraged to live in village communities near the hospital. Traditional healers worked as a team in consultation with the hospital doctors. Dr. Lambo believes that traditional healing methods, which often include confession, dancing, rituals, features inherent in traditional cults, together with the tolerance in the village environment, are positive elements for healing and should be utilized. Lambo shows the social therapeutic and economic advantages of keeping mental patients in a traditional village community, but he does not touch upon the problem of sorcery, witchcraft and non-scientific beliefs that arise if the healing practices of the traditional mganga are accepted as part of the cure.

Western psychiatry must learn to make more creative use of traditional culture and healing practices if it wishes to increase its therapeutic care and rehabilitation of the mentally ill. As it is, the mentally ill continue to have local medicine smuggled into the hospitals. G. Jahoda of Ghana, who has written much on the importance of traditional medicine in African psychiatry, points out: "the lesson is that any campaign of enlightenment ought to be cautious in condemning traditional healers and similar institutions because they perform an extremely important social function." (Jahoda, 1961) Raymond Prince, who has studied indigenous Yoruba psychiatry, differentiates between recommending indigenous physical healing practices and recommending psychological therapy. He states:[3]

> "It seems clear that there is no good reason to encourage indigenous healing practices for physical illness in any culture. Western diagnostic technique and western pharmacological and surgical knowledge far outstrip every other known system of medicine. In addition, western practices are universally applicable: they are not culture-bound. Psychological medicine is different, however, in a number of ways. Western psychiatric techniques are not in my opinion demonstrably superior to many indigenous Yoruba practices. Psychotherapeutic techniques fit the cultures in which they have developed and cannot cross cultural boundaries so successfully as can physical therapies." (Prince, 1964, 116)

As for "Western" superiority in techniques for physical healing, we might well be reminded today that "Eastern" Chinese acupuncture seems to offer a new approach from which medical science is trying to learn. As for psychotherapy, most writers agree with Lambo when he writes: "We have repeatedly found that in the sphere of psychoneuroses some illiterate patients who have failed to respond to our kind of approach have recovered under the influence of native psychotherapists at the native treatment centres." (Lambo quoted in Prince, 1964, 116)

c. *Marital Problems*:

Seven problems of marriage were amongst the 100 cases. Six of these involved accusations of sorcery. Jealousy and unfaithfulness appear to give rise to accusations of sorcery between husbands and wives and suspected lovers. In five cases bodily illness was the basis for sorcery accusation. If a woman loses the cloth she keeps for her menstrual period it is immediately assumed that someone has stolen it in order to bewitch her or to make her barren. In one case the sister of the client's husband was accused of stealing the client's cloth because she hated her and wanted her to leave her brother.

In another case the wife had refused her husband sexual relations, impelling him to take her cloth and treat it with *uchawi* in order to make her sick.

Polygamy also gives rise to tension between wives. In one case here the second wife had a child, creating jealousy and subsequent accusations from the first wife. Such tension was evident also in a case involving a mentally ill woman and the second wife of her husband. More often, however, sorcery is used as grounds for divorcing the accused or for ousting one spouse in order to remarry.

A one-eyed cat was thought to have been sent into a wife's kitchen by her husband's lover, to drive her away. The wife went to a mganga first for protection and afterwards to arrange a divorce. Another wife refused her husband sexual relations because he did not provide her with clothes or money. Later she accused him of sorcery and wanted a divorce. In a different case it was the wife who bewitched the husband in order to leave him for another man.

Only one marital case brought to a mganga did not involve sorcery. In this case, the husband was jealous of his wife's friends and accused her of unfaithfulness. Because of his jealousy he beat her often and frequently accused her unjustly. Feeling sorry for the wife, a woman living in the same house arranged for her brother, a *shehe*, to visit the wife secretly during her husband's absence. This rendezvous resulted in a secret love affair between the wife and the *shehe*. On the occasion of another beating, the wife suggested to her husband that they call in their neighbor's *shehe* brother and ask him to read an *Amini*, Sw. The *Amini* is an Islamic oath of faithfulness which is believed to have the power of death over an unfaithful spouse.

The *shehe*, knowing the plot to teach the husband a lesson, agreed to administer the *Amini* oath to this husband and wife. They were given water for a purification wash; then they sat on a mat and the *shehe* read many portions from the Koran. *Ubani* was burnt, and finally the oath was taken: "If I go out with another man/woman, let the *Amini* kill me." They paid the *shehe* 15 shillings for the rite.

After this the husband trusted his wife and stopped beating her, he himself remaining faithful to her. But the wife and the *shehe*, amused by the husband's gullibility, continued as secret lovers.

Of the six marital cases involving sorcery, four had been taken to a diviner, one was unknown, and one client said she had not gone to a diviner. In the Zaramo Muslim society where marital quarrels and divorce have become an expected though unpleasant experience, it appears that the diviners/waganga capitalize on the situation. Rather than acting as peacemakers and preservers of the marital code which traditionally disapproves of divorce, they support the accusations and fears of sorcery between husband and wife. Because people experience expressions of hatred, jealousy and unfaithfulness in their daily lives and believe that sorcery can cause illness and misfortune, they are ready to believe the waganga's confirmation of this. If the Zaramo's suspicions were not continually encouraged by the *ramli* verdict of the waganga, accusations of sorcery over marital problems might easily decrease.

d. *Business Problems*:
In traditional rural society the waganga have had a profitable business protecting their client's crops and property from theft and destruction by evildoers. Also it has been the mganga's task to treat the seeds and fields for fertility and to assure an abundant harvest. Today the urban mganga has no seeds or *shambas*, fields, to treat but offer power for the protection and success of business.

Among the 63 sorcery cases, three involved unsuccessful businesses. The three clients were men operating small provisions shops. Their cases were very similar in that their business was declining and two of the men were physically ill. One of the clients suspected that someone had put a *jini* in his shop to drive away customers.

All three clients contended that their misfortune was caused by jealous neighbors who wished to ruin their good business. All three had gone first to a diviner and therefore were convinced that neighbors had used sorcery against them. One client had not only received *dawa* for his illness, and to counteract the power of sorcery, but also had taken steps for revenge. He was one of the few clients who admitted having gone to a mganga for *uchawi*. He declared that the person who had used sorcery against him would die because of it: "People won't play tricks on me anymore, and if they do they themselves will be harmed."

The task of the waganga in these three cases was to counteract the power of sorcery, to heal the clients' physical ills, and to restore their businesses. Had the waganga understood the economics of good retailing business they might have made suggestions to their clients on selling different lines of goods or improving their salesmanship and advertising. Instead, their diagnoses of the problems were to blame someone else, thus perpetuating and even promoting community tension. The end result might be even further loss of business due to continued accusations and fear of revenge.

e. *Misfortune*:
Almost any event of misfortune is assumed by the Zaramo to be the work of sorcery. This was apparent in the cases of the three failing business enterprises and even physical illness might be considered as misfortune.

Rashidi, a boy about nine years old, was walking across an empty lot in Temeke one morning when he was bitten by a poisonous snake. The father rushed his son to a local medicine man for treatment, and then in the evening went to a diviner to learn the cause of this misfortune. He himself suspected that his son had been bewitched. He reasoned that because the misfortune had occurred in the daylight and in a very open place, someone must have sent the snake to attack the boy. Therefore he did not take the boy to a hospital.

The diviner confirmed the father's suspicions of *uchawi*, adding that if the father had taken his son to a hospital the boy would have died. When asked if he wished to take revenge on the bewitcher, the father replied that he would wait until his son recovered and then decide.

Regardless of whether misfortune comes in the form of a snake bite, a car accident, or a broken arm or leg, the mganga reaffirms the belief that accidents do not just happen, but that all unfortunate events have a cause and that the cause is nearly always the work of sorcery. I do not doubt that the mganga himself is sincere in this belief. The fact that he can treat a snake bite successfully is commendable, but his real profit in the business comes when he treats the victim for sorcery and charges another 40 shillings for a protection amulet.

Another example of misfortune ascribed to sorcery is illustrated in the case of Naval Seaman C.B., who was one of forty Tanzanians sent to the Soviet Union for two years to be trained for the new Tanzanian Navy. Seaman C.B. returned to Tanzania after successfully completing his course in radio communications. Because the Navy was at that time without its own quarters, the forty men were housed in the Army's Colito Barracks in Dar es Salaam.

Shortly after the Navy men had settled into the Army quarters two of the men died in scooter accidents and one man died in a car accident. The sailor had suspected that the older Army men were jealous of the Navy, and now this opinion was being confirmed; the sailors were being bewitched and killed. Two sailors resigned immediately in fear of their lives.

Seaman C.B. was very worried that he also would be killed and went to his brother to confide this fear, enquiring also about a good Swahili mganga who could give him protection medicine. The brother tried to convince C.B. that such medicines were useless and that sorcery was only in one's imagination.

But Seaman C.B. was not convinced by his brother, and approached his step-father, who agreed to help him. The step-father first consulted a mganga in the Tandika/Temeke area to have the situation divined. Yes, said the mganga, the seaman is being bewitched and must have protection medicine. He asked the step-father to bring his son immediately so that he might protect him. The medicine would cost 160 shillings, but this, he consoled, was really a very small amount considering that the son was still young. The mganga said he really only wanted to help him, and added further that this medicine would even stop bullets in time of war.

When Seaman C.B. heard that the medicine would stop bullets in time of war he laughed, recognizing the ridiculousness of such an assertion. He said that he could no longer believe that mganga. Nevertheless, Seaman C.B. did not lose his fear, and consequently left the naval service, together with most of his companions. Thereby, what was probably the first Tanzanian naval unit was soon disbanded (or it might be said that it went down defeated by the fears and accusations of sorcery).

As a footnote to this case it should be explained that after returning from the USSR most of the forty men received between one and two thousand shillings in back pay. With this money, some bought scooters or cars, and went in for a gay life. All three accidents occurred as the men were returning from a drinking club. The verdict in the newspapers was death due to drunken driving, but the verdict of the waganga, and of popular belief, was death due to bewitching by jealous Army men. In both the case of the boy bitten by a snake and the defeated Navy men, it was the diviner/mganga who fostered the belief that their misfortune had its source in the evil intent of other men.

3. Protection

Fear of sorcery compels thousands of Zaramo to take protective measures either to prevent bewitching or to avoid repetition of illness or misfortune which has already occurred. The providing of protection was ranked third amongst the services administered by the 60 waganga interviewed. A day's case load included as many as 120 clients in need of protection medicine.

In the 100 case studies I found only four clients who listed their problem as that of seeking protection. I have explained previously how protection is normally considered a part of the treatment for sorcery and therefore it is generally listed under that category rather than under protection. Of the 63 cases involving sorcery the majority of clients mentioned that they would be taking or had already taken protective medicine. The following five cases, however, illustrate the situations in which only protection was sought.

Fear is the basic factor leading people to seek protection. If you believe it is possible for other persons to harm you through magical or real poisons, if you see daily evidence of such practices in the society around you, if you have suspicion and the fear that someone is trying to bewitch you, then it is only common sense that you should take precautionary measures. This thinking is as logical to the vast majority of Zaramo as that which leads to vaccination against the dangers of smallpox and polio. What mother would allow her child to get sick or die when for a few shillings she can buy a *hirizi* to ward off the evil spirits and evildoers ?

A woman who owned a house in Kariakoo was building a new one in Manzese. She had had some unpleasant experiences with the tenants in her current home and wanted to avoid such troubles with her new tenants. Therefore she went to a mganga, *fundi wa kitabu*, "specialist of the book", to have a *halubadili* read before the tenants moved into the new house. This assured her that the tenants would pay their rent regularly and not cause trouble or bewitch her. If they did commit any evil against her they themselves would suffer through sickness or death. The woman said that she would warn the new tenants beforehand so that they would be afraid to cause her any ill-will.

The second case also involved the seeking of protection through the reading of the *halubadili.* This woman, named Asha, had only a general fear of sorcery and felt she should be protected against the possibility of attack. Therefore she went to a Muslim *mwalimu* to have the *halubadili* read. The *mwalimu* and client sat on a mat before a charcoal fire and empty clay pot as the *mwalimu* declared : "I am going to read the *halubadili* and if any one thinks of doing bad things to you he will die. If any person wants to give you *uchawi* he will die. So don't be afraid; you can go anywhere. No *jini* or anything bad shall touch you."

After chanting several portions of the Koran the *mwalimu* placed the clay pot on the charcoal fire, putting salt, coffee beans and seven sewing needles inside the pot. He then continued : "If anyone wants to do a bad thing to Asha, he or she must die; no bad thing shall touch her." Asha was asked to recite similar words. After chanting more verses from the Koran the *mwalimu* instructed Asha to pour a bowlful of water into the clay pot while he repeated the curse for the third time. "If anyone wants to do evil to you let him die." The entire ritual lasted about 40 minutes and the charge was 40 shillings.

The young man in the third case was employed as a cashier in a canteen. He feared that his fellow workers might steal money from the cash register or cause him to lose his job through sorcery. He determined to prevent such an eventuality by using protective medicine which he sought from a mganga in Buguruni.

As the client sat on a floor mat in front of the mganga a dead lizard tied to a board was placed in his lap. The mganga proceeded to read the Koran in Arabic for about 40 minutes. After the reading they went together to a nearby field to bury the lizard.

Although the client did not understand Arabic, he knew that a curse was being read and that this curse would harm anyone who tried to bewitch him. The mganga told him not to eat or drink anything which was left over by another person. Should he violate this rule the medicine would lose its power.

The next day the client returned to the mganga to obtain an amulet which contained written verses from the *halubadili.* The man thereafter carried the amulet to work and sometimes put it under the seat of his stool at the cashier's counter.

In the forth case, a Zaramo woman had been having a secret love affair while married to an Arab. When she decided to terminate her illicit sexual relations she discovered that her menstruation cloth was missing. She suspected that her lover had stolen it in order to harm her or to make her barren. In an effort to counteract this possibility she went to a mganga for protection and he in turn recommended that she go to a *mwalimu wa kitabu* for a *halubadili* reading. But when she said she preferred not to go to another "practitioner", the mganga agreed to protect her with local medicine.

The fifth case has been described already under the category of misfortune. In short, when three Navy men died in road accidents which were ascribed to the work of sorcery by jealous Army men, a Seaman, fearing that he also would be bewitched by the Army men, sought protective medicine.

In all five cases no harm had actually been experienced by the clients themselves. It was the *fear* of harm which led them to the waganga. In these cases we see the role of the mganga as that of defender, protector and comforter.

Providing protection is a relatively easy procedure, with few risks involved. Within these five cases the cheapest *halubadili* reading cost only 40 shillings while the most expensive treatment offered was priced at 160 shillings.

In eleven cases in which protection was sought after *uchawi* had been already detected and the misfortune treated, the average charge was 123 shillings. If a client simply bought an amulet as prevention against *uchawi* the average cost was 46 shillings. In most cases the protection costs were higher than the cure for illness. Protective measures are considered most effective when performed by recognized specialists, and people are willing to pay more accordingly. The *halubadili* is generally read by a *shehe* or *mwalimu* whose professional fees are appropriately higher than those of the ordinary mganga. The *shehe* or *mwalimu's* religious role of "priest" in the sense of Muslim cleric enhances his position and power, giving confidence in God's readiness to intervene in case of *uchawi.*

Although Zaramo Christians are sometimes fearful of sorcery and will seek protection when troubled, it is noticeable that in non-Muslim areas of Tanzania where Christianity has been the dominant religious force for several generations, the fear of sorcery and the use of amulets has become less frequent. The seeking of protection against sorcery remains a practice primarily in Muslim society and amongst those people who have retained their traditional religious beliefs.

Roman Catholic theology and teaching in Tanzania has changed significantly with regard to the wearing of crosses and the medals of saints for protection, but the average Tanzanian Christian probably continues to wear a medal for the same reason that a non-Christian may wear a Koranic or herbal *hirizi.* The Zaramo Lutheran who does not have access to such medals of saints may continue to rely upon the more traditional or Muslim protective medicine.

As long as the Zaramo are not free from the fear of sorcery and as long waganga continue to attribute illness and misfortune to acts of sorcery, the sale of amulets will persist and the waganga will flourish in their role as protectors and defenders of innocent people against evildoers.

4. Spirits and Ritual Obligations

Three other categories of special problems dealt with by the medicine men did not entertain the thought of sorcery but of ancestor spirits and other traditional beliefs. Of the 100 Zaramo studied, ten concerned spirit beliefs and ritual obligations. Five concerned unemployed men who were involved in court and theft cases .

Six problems presented in the ten spirit and ritual obligation cases (See Table 6) consisted of physical ailments. Only stomach troubles and a rash on the leg were specified. Three problems were apparently psychic disturbances; a screaming fit, a dancing fit, and a state of trance. One case which might seem to be mis-categorized was that of a palm-wine seller whose business was failing.

Four of the ten clients stated that they had gone first to a hospital or clinic for treatment but that the treatment failed to help them. One man recounted that he had been admitted to a hospital because of unbearable aching in his legs. When he felt no relief by the fifth day the doctors reportedly told him to go home to his parents for treatment.

It is apparent that some medical personnel in Dar es Salaam hospitals and dispensaries at times recommend treatment by traditional medicine men. If a problem cannot be diagnosed by the medical staff in the hospital and if patients insist that they have been bewitched or are possessed by a spirit, there may be no alternative but to discharge them. In such circumstances it is unlikely that a patient will respond to modern cures.

TABLE 6: Spirits and Ritual Obligations

Data from 10 Cases

Case No.	Sex	Divier used?	Symptom of problem	Cause	Relationship	Did client go first to Gov't Hospital for treatment?
S.3	F	Yes	Stomach trouble	Neglected ancestor spirit grave	Mother's spirit grave	Yes. Went to dispensary for 3 days. They can't cure this kind of trouble.
S.11	F	Yes	Whole body sick	Neglected ancestor's grave	Father's father's spirit	Yes. For one month. Then made *tambiko*.
S.27	F	Yes	Sick for six months	Kinyamkera spirit possession	Belongs to Kinyamkera	No. Children tried to take her but she would not go.
S.31	M	No	Rash on leg	He had broken his taboo and must make *tambiko* at grave.	Mother's father's grave	Yes. Admitted to hospital for 5 days. He was told by doctor to go to mganga; cured in 2 days.
S.62	M	Yes	Palm-wine selling business declining	Neglected mother's mother's grave	Ancestor spirit	No. Went to a diviner who told him of his neglect. He had to make *tambiko* and ask for forgiveness.
S.85	F	Yes	Very sick	Neglected ancestor spirit. Had to make *tambiko* at grave.	Grave of oldest male ancestor in family	Yes. Went to hospital for 4 days. Was discharged still ill. Mganga advised *tambiko*; cured in 4 days.
S.93	M	Yes	Six month old baby continually cried	Needed to have its grandfather's name. Parents had neglected *jadi*	Ancestor spirit of father.	No. Went to mganga who said baby needed grandfather's name.
S.95	F	No	Lonely woman began screaming.	The spirit wants attention. Taken by spirit. Needs *sadaka*		No. Went to *shehe* to have Koran read for exorcism of the spirit.
S.96	F	?	Woman went into trance for 3 days. Eyes open but not breathing.	Spirit possession.	Spirit adept	No. Special mganga from Bagamoyo called in. Worked two days to free her.
S.100	F	Yes	Wife went into dancing fit. Husband became sick when he beat her.	*Ashetani* spirit possessed her. She had to dance the *kiluwa*	Spirit *shetani*	No. Went to mganga for divining and spirit medicine. She was told to dance.

I recorded only one statement by a Tanzanian Medical Assistant working in a Dar es Salaam hospital, but his view of local medicines may be fairly typical of the thinking of medical personnel from the coastal area.

Medical Assistant N.K., when asked if local medicines are effective, replied:

> "Yes, very much, and you must not despise them. There are diseases which cannot be treated in hospitals. Some sicknesses cannot be cured unless one uses local *dawa*. I myself once suffered from stomach troubles and no medicine from the hospital helped me. I then used local medicine for almost two weeks and was cured. Since then I have not had stomach trouble again. I do not believe that people who have been bewitched can be helped by hospital medicine; they must apply local *dawa*."

The same Medical Assistant said he did not believe there was medicine which could bring good luck, such as for passing examinations or for winning in gambling. But his belief in local *dawa* to counteract sorcery and some types of illness would be affirmed by many hospital workers. Three of the 100 clients being treated by waganga were in fact hospital staff members, one being a nurse.

Of these ten spirit and ritual obligation cases, seven involved neglect of the family ancestor spirit. Most of these clients admitted to having been delinquent about making the yearly *tambiko*, ritual offering, at a particular grave, such as the spirit grave of the mother, the father's father, the mother's father, or of the eldest male ancestor spirit.

Another specific ancestor spirit case was that of a mother who neglected to name her baby after the father's father. In this case the young baby cried continually. When the father consulted a mganga for *ramli* to find out the cause of crying, he was told that the baby was crying for his grandfather's name. The ancestor spirit had been angered by the parents' misnaming of their child and was therefore disturbing the baby.

Accepting the mganga's assessment of the problem, the father and mother took their baby to a rubbish heap and deposited him on it. To the Zaramo a rubbish heap is a symbol of death and no doubt was used in this rite to signify that the child was now dead and would be born afresh with a new name. Proceeding with the rite, the mother took a mouthful of water from a *kata*, a ladle used for drinking, and spat it into the mouth of the baby. Having done this, she gave in the Zaramo language the following pledge: *"Lelo vino mwana yuno tomgwelela ditagwa juulondile diyolela yolilia avo kokemwa Nmyamani kama gwegwe"* , (Today this son is given the name he has been crying for and he is called Mnyamani as you were called).

Spitting into the mouth of a new-born baby is a Zaramo ritual signifying that the child is now of the same human spirit as his parents. In this above - mentioned case the child was treated as a new-born baby in order to undo the mistake made earlier. The mother explained later: "If we hadn't given him the name Mnyamani he would not have stopped crying and in the end would have become sick and possibly died."

The remaining four cases had to do with spirit possession.The elderly woman in Case S.27 stated in agreement with a diviner that she was possessed by the Kinyamkera spirit. Her children wanted to take her to hospital, as she had been ill for six months despite repeated treatment by local waganga, but she refused to go. Instead she visited a diviner and was told of being possessed by the spirit Kinyamkera. Her children arranged to have a *madogoli*, exorcism, performed for their mother, but this didn't restore her health. Finally, in desperation the children attempted to deceive their mother into going to the Kigamboni dispensary. On the way to the dispensary she suddenly realized what her children were doing to her. She sat down in the middle of the road and cried: "You are tired of me now, that is why you take me to the hospital. It is only Kinyamkera but you are not looking for the right mganga. If I go to the hospital Kinyamkera will be very angry and she will kill me because she does not get her *sadaka* , offering." In the end the children were obliged to take their mother back home.

Case S.95 concerned a woman who thought herself possessed by a *shetani* spirit and who had shut herself in a room for a week. When she suddenly began screaming, crying and trembling the neighbors rushed in and grabbed her by the ear, asking the spirit what it wanted. Eventually the spirit answered through the stifled voice of the woman, as is customary. She said she was not sick, but that her *shetani* spirit did not like people and caused her to hate even her husband. The husband was told that he must take his wife to a *shehe* to have the Koran read over his wife. This he did the following day. The spirit which had possessed his wife was thought to be Mwenembago, a well-known Zaramo spirit.

Case S.96 was that of a woman who went into a state of trance for a period of three days. Her eyes were wide open, her heart was beating, but the husband and neighbors could not detect any breathing. On the third night the neighbors were awakened by the husband reporting that his wife was very sick. The woman was found sitting with her eyes open but otherwise appearing as if dead. One man suggested that her eyes should be closed and the corpse prepared for a burial. The relatives arrived shortly and recognized that the woman was not dead but in a state of trance. They believed she had been possessed by a *shetani*.

A special mganga was summoned from Bagamoyo to treat her in Dar es Salaam. The relatives later reported : "He had to work two days before he managed to make her breathe and speak." Once she had recovered from the trance she was as strong and normal as before the problem occurred.

Hadija, in Case S.100, was said to be possessed by a *shetani* which compelled her to dance the *kiluwa*. Those who witnessed her dancing said that she danced as though possessed by a spirit or in a state of trance. Her husband returned home one day and found her dancing this *ngoma*, the *kiluwa*, nearby, with a group of people. Strongly disapproving of such behavior he beat her and forced her to go home, where he continued to beat her. But the wife continued her dancing as though completely unaware of what she was doing.

The next morning the husband awakened to find his entire body swollen. He was taken to the hospital but could not be helped. His relatives then went to a diviner and were told that the man's body had become swollen because he had punished his wife for dancing *kiluwa*. The diviner explained that she had not danced of her own accord but was driven to do so by a *shetani*. Now if this man wished to recover from the swelling he must allow his wife to go on dancing, but come himself to the mganga for treatment. The informant added wryly : "That wife is good *kiluwa* dancer up to this day!"

It is not the intention of this study to judge the credibility of these accounts, such as whether or not a *shetani* possessed this particular woman and made her dance or whether the woman in Case S.96 did or did not breathe for three to five days. The basic concern is what people believe to happen and what role the waganga/diviners play in moulding Zaramo opinion. In these three cases the waganga are seen again as preservers of Zaramo traditional belief in the work and power of spirits. Kinyamkera and Mwenembago were once more affirmed in the life of the community. The mganga in Case S.100 actually sanctioned the work of the *shetani* by judging the husband guilty of interfering by trying to stop his wife's dancing fit, and warning him of continued illness if he did not desist. In their divination and treatments waganga either tacitly or openly advise respect and obedience toward ancestor spirits and other general or particular spirits.

These ten spirit cases reflect a changing pattern in the work of urban waganga. They represent only 10 per cent of the total of 100 Zaramo cases recorded. In one day's total case load of the 60 waganga only two spirit cases were reported out of a total of 636 cases. Possibly there were other cases recorded as sickness treatments, but even so not more than one per cent of their cases involved spirits or ritual obligations. This is in sharp contrast to the work of rural Zaramo waganga, the majority of whose cases involve calamity or illness believed to be caused by spirit intervention. Only a lesser number of such cases are ascribed to *uchawi*.

M-L. Swantz (1970, 133) recorded 62 cases of divination in a Zaramo rural area, and divided the causes given at divination into three major categories. I did the same with my 100 urban Zaramo cases, for purposes of comparison. The results indicated significant changes taking place in the urban Zaramo society. In the rural area study the majority (58%) of illness and misfortune cases were said by the diviner to be caused by the intervention of spirits. This is in sharp contrast to the urban cases, where only 10 per cent were found to be spirit cases. Some explanation for this must be offered.

Spirit cases are generally treated either by exorcism rites, *madogoli*, or by the client's making a ritual offering, *tambiko*, to the spirit. If such treatment were suggested by the urban mganga he would lose his client. If an exorcism were to be performed it would have to be done by a mganga of the particular spirit possessing the client. The client would normally go back to the rural "home" village where the ancestor's grave or spirit hut is located to perform the ritual offering. In either case the urban mganga would lose his client. At best he could suggest taking some spirit medicine first and then going to make the *tambiko* for the spirit. In this case his financial gain would be very small.

It should be stated also that the urban environment does not lend itself to the performance of spirit exorcism. A fairly large space is needed for the performance of dancing and drumming which normally takes a full night and a day. All of the client's extended family are expected to take part, which could cause a housing and feeding problem if located in the city. Then, too, the noise of the drums and singing would cause a disturbance of the peace and sleep of the city dwellers. In view of this it is much easier for the urban mganga to suggest sorcery as the cause rather than spirit activity.

The urban mganga capitalizes on the tensions he knows to exist between neighbors and co-workers in a crowded city. These fears and tensions are ready material for accusations of sorcery. While the rural waganga at Bunju ascribed 27.5 per cent of the causes of calamity and illness to sorcery, the urban waganga in my 100 cases attributed 63 per cent to sorcery. Sorcery cases are relatively simple to treat compared with the work involved in exorcism, and are more profitable. This marked change in the explanation for the cause of the problem serves to substantiate my hypothesis that the new urban social environment, with its accompanying tensions, allows a new set of accusations to be proposed as an explanation for the cause of illness and misfortune.

5. Work/Unemployment

A serious unemployment problem has become a characteristic of most rapidly-growing African cities. Dar es Salaam is no exception. The rate of migration into the city far exceeds the development of job opportunities, making unemployment a constant feature. Because the Zaramo people have been well-established in Dar es Salaam for the past hundred years, nearly all rural Zaramo have some family or clan member in the city. Thus being assured of a place to stay while seeking a job, nearly every young Zaramo man comes to the city at some time or other to take his chance in seeking employment.

Then a mganga who has traditionally performed the role of agriculturalist in providing fertility *dawa* for seeds and assuring protection of good harvest for crops, must now make his service relevant to the urban situation. His altered, modernized role has become chiefly that of aiding men in securing employment, in earning promotion, or in simply keeping a job.

Five cases out of the 100 Zaramo cases studied dealt with unemployment problems. Amongst these, however, none involved the matter of promotion or job security.

Four said they had gone first to a diviner to learn the cause of their unemployment. Two clients were advised of bad fortune in their bodies which had to be removed. This was to be done by a cleansing or purification process.

In two cases the spirits had been angered by neglect and therefore caused unemployment. In case S.89 the man had forgotten his *jadi*, neglecting to make *tambiko* at the *mkungu*, spirit hut. In Case S.91 the man had neglected his mother's mother's grave and it was her spirit which was angry.

In Case S.88 the unemployed man had been given amulets to wear, medicine in which to bathe and other medicine to chew, but he was not helped. He concluded that medicines were useless and that acquiring a job really depended on luck and popularity. His final comment, however, betrayed a belief in some type of outside force. "If parents are angry, one might not get a job. Parents are like a second God and one may not get a job if disobedient to them."

For all five men the waganga not only recommended the keeping of the ritual obligation at the spirit grave and the ritualistic outward cleansing of the body, but also prescribed work medicines for internal use. This was in recognition that the problem was not due to external forces, but was also rooted in neglect by the client. Thus the necessity for inner purification.

S.87 was given medicine in which to bathe as well as to eat and to place under his pillow. S.88 obtained medicine for bathing, for chewing and for wearing. S.89 made a *tambiko* and took medicine internally. S.91 also made a *tambiko* and was given medicine in which to bathe, but in addition he was given leaves to burn in order to be cleansed by the smoke and he purchased a *hirizi* to carry in his pocket. S.92 took only external cleansing medicine.

Were the clients satisfied with the results reportedly effected by these work medicines and *jadi* cures? It seems so. One man who had been unemployed for four years secured a job within two weeks. Another man out of work for four years was employed as a driver within a month. The man who made an offering at his mother's mother's grave got a job as a driver very shortly afterwards. It seems that in all but Case S.88 the clients were pleased with the results of the treatment received and were convinced that it was this medicine which changed their situations

In addition to these five specific cases of unemployed men, eight other Zaramo men were interviewed at random regarding their opinion on the effectiveness of work medicines. The sample is small but indicates a relatively consistent way of thinking.

When asked : "Do people in this city go to waganga for medicine to help them get jobs ?", all eight affirmed that this was common. They implied that it was a generally acceptable practice, especially amongst the Muslims. Three stated that the Muslim *shehe* and *mwalimu* supplied the best medicine for employment. When asked : "Have you yourselves ever bought medicine for getting work ?" three answered that they had done so, and five said no. The question was then re-phrased : "Do you think this sort of medicine really works ?" Five replied that they believed it was effective and three stated that they did not place any faith in such *dawa* or amulets.

This sample is too small to be used as an accurate measurement of Zaramo opinion or practice, but when paralleled with the estimates provided by the waganga it has some merit. When confronted with modern urban problems, the mganga relies upon traditional beliefs and magical skills, but revises his methods to accommodate the uniqueness of present-day circumstances. In this sense he is both the innovator and preserver of tradition.

6. Crime and Legal Cases

In the pre-colonial days the Zaramo people enforced their own community moral code and dealt with offenders through several recognized channels of authority. The headman of the village, known as a *m'hadsi* or *mpazi*, Z., or *mdewa*, Sw., was the highest authority. The *m'hadsi*, together with a group of elders or counselors, constituted the local authority and all disputes could be brought to them for settlement. For more serious cases such as sorcery accusations, in which the verdict meant death for the guilty, local courts, *kitala*, Sw., with authorized judges, *wasemi*, and advocates, *wakalangama*, for the accused were assembled to determine the verdict. After the verdict was announced, it was the clan members of the guilty victim who carried out the death sentence, often by burning the accused.

As an alternative method of judging a case, the suspected party was brought before a mganga/ diviner for an ordeal. Twelve different types of Zaramo ordeals have been described in *The Zaramo of Tanzania* (L.W. Swantz 1966, 61-62). In some cases the ordeal itself was certain to affirm the accusation and punish the victim simultaneously as he was forced to insert his hand in boiling water, walk seven times across glowing hot iron, or drink poison.

Today such courts have been replaced by local government courts and magistrates and by the legal system of the country. Traditional waganga do not have the legal authority to try suspected offenders nor to accuse specific persons of being witches or sorcerers. Nor it is legal to punish an accused person through ordeals. To do so would be contrary to the present law of the land and the mganga himself would be liable to court fines or imprisonment.

The waganga in Dar es Salaam, however, do participate in the present legal and judicial system at least indirectly. They may not accuse a person of guilt, but the guilty frequently reveal themselves and confess. Furthermore, the waganga do not openly contest or prejudice the judge and court, but by their insinuations and magic it is believed that they can change or influence the decision of the judge or accusers. The following court, prison and theft cases disclose how the urban Zaramo mganga plays indirectly the role of judge and advocate.

Three cases involved theft. In the first case, S.38, someone had broken into the client's house and stolen 1,600 shillings, a watch and several gold rings. The owner reported the theft to the police and then went to a diviner to enquire who was guilty. His daughter meanwhile went to a *shehe* for a reading of the *halubadili* to ensure that if the thief did not return the money he would die.

The diviner revealed that the person who stole the money and other items was a relative of the owner and that he had not yet used the money but was waiting to see what would happen. In this case, as in all others included in this study, the diviner never revealed the guilty person by name. In this respect the diviner keeps within the law. Mganga Matoroka, the itinerant witch-finder described earlier, explained that the verdict rests on the outcome of the medicine treatment. If a person is guilty and does not change his ways, he will die or become seriously ill. This method of leaving the outcome to self-accusation or self-revelation of guilt is illustrated in the following case.

Three Zaramo prostitutes rented a single room to carry on their business during the daytime, while at night each returned to her regular partner. One evening one of these women left 60 shillings under her pillow before leaving for her own home. When she returned to the room in the morning she found her money missing and her two friends denied any knowledge of it.

The owner of the house was summoned and it was agreed that they call a mganga to perform an ordeal for testing the innocence or guilt of everyone living in the house. When the mganga came one evening all occupants of the house were assembled together before a plate of rice. The mganga asked each person to come forward and take one grain of rice, putting it into his or her mouth. In so doing the guilty person would be revealed shortly.

Each person followed the mganga's instructions. Before long one woman's mouth was completely full of rice so that she could not contain it at all. When questioned she admitted having taken the money. She was a married woman and was severely beaten by her husband after this incident.

The woman informant in this case was one of the occupants of the house and had gone through the ordeal herself. She claimed to have seen the rice flow from the accused's mouth. Here the mganga did not need to accuse or punish anyone, for the guilty woman revealed herself in the course of the ordeal and her husband took it upon himself to administer the punishment.

In Case S.40 a possibly innocent boy was made to suffer. Ramadhani, a very young man, had rented a room in Mtoni. One night someone tried to break into the room of the owner of the house, but the owner woke up before the thief had a chance to take anything. The thief ran away and the owner later suspected that the shoe marks left behind were those of the youth Ramadhani.

To confirm his suspicion the owner went to a mganga for *ramli*. The divination revealed that three shillings had been taken from the top of the table. Although the owner knew that this was not true, as the thief had not succeeded in entering the room, he determined to seek revenge against Ramadhani.

When Ramadhani heard this he moved to another part of Dar es Salaam for fear of being bewitched. Such accusations, the fear of revenge or the assumption that real sickness and misfortune are due to sorcery, account for the high proportion of Dar es Salaam residents who shift to new living quarters each year. The mganga in his role of judge and revealer of crime tends to heighten social tension rather than alleviate fears.

Case S.49 had been sentenced to prison for theft. His brother and some other relatives visited a mganga with the hope of altering the prison sentence. The mganga instructed the prisoner's relatives to purchase a white goat to be buried alive. They were instructed further to build a fire on the ground above the buried goat and cook medicines for the release of the prisoner.

After the medicine had been thus prepared the fire was extinguished and the goat was dug out from the ground. According to the mganga, if the goat had died the man would remain in prison, but if the goat was still alive the man would be released shortly. In this case the goat was still alive and the brother returned home from prison within two weeks. The goat was taken by the mganga as payment together with 150 shillings in cash.

Case S.50 was not so fortunate. While employed in Government service, this man had accepted a bribe of 55 shillings. In an effort to procure acquittal in the trial the man and his parents spent much money buying *dawa* from various medicine men. The accused was given an amulet which he was to carry around the court house the night before the trial and other medicine to be chewed during the trial. Despite all these efforts he was sentenced to two years imprisonment plus 24 strokes.

Ali, Case S.51, had a similar result, only his medicines were more elaborate. They included a boiled chicken cooked together with roots, stones, bells and ropes. Before eating this *dawa*, he had to sit under a three colored cloth, in the steam of the chicken-soup pot, for vapor treatment. Furthermore, three pieces of wood tied inside a handkerchief were to be carried into the courtroom. When asked about the end result of all this, the man replied solemnly: "Sad news, I went to prison."

To win his theft case, S.52 was given *madawa* to drink. The mganga whom he had consulted wrote words from the Koran with colored ink on a plate. The plate was then rinsed with water which the client drank afterwards. More words from the Koran were written on blue paper and sewn inside white cloth as an amulet for him to carry into the court room. Another small white amulet was provided for keeping in his mouth during the court proceedings. The price for the amulets was 40 shillings. In this case the outcome was not disclosed.

Six additional interviews on this subject were carried out, confirming the fact that Zaramo people generally consult a mganga when in difficulty with the law. The waganga have successfully convinced the Zaramo public that their medicines are above the law and can affect the judge's verdict or alter a prison sentence. Although the mganga still fulfils the traditional role of witch-finder and revealer of thieves, he has now modernized his post to that of defendant or "office for special appeals". This latter position is more attractive than the former, for anti-witch *dawa* costs only 60 cents per adult, whereas a good court case might enrich the mganga by 100 shillings.

7. Sexual Problems

The sixty waganga in this study ranked sexual problems fifth in the number of cases brought to them. In the actual case loads of the previous day, however, only two cases were reported out of a total of 636 clients treated, and in the 100 client study only one case was found. Six cases were reported by the waganga as being treated on the day of the interviews, which indicates more attention to sexual problems than the figures in my completed interviews imply. Although the general public may have a keen interest in sexual problems and the help which traditional waganga can give, in actual fact the mganga spends relatively little time treating such problems. When interviewing Zaramo on this topic, endless information was given but it did not correspond to the specific problems brought to the mganga's waiting room.

It is true that in the cases concerned with marital problems there were two which involved quarrels about sexual relations between husband and wife, and three accusations of unfaithfulness in sexual relations. Also in the sorcery and protection cases there were several women who believed their menstrual cloths had been stolen or that excessive bleeding was being caused by someone trying to make them barren. In this particular category, however, I have limited the examples to only those problems which relate directly to the physical act of sexual intercourse or the procreation of children.

The only such case found in this study was that of a young married couple who had recently become parents for the first time. The couple wished to resume normal sexual relations but believed that if they did so before their baby was weaned it would become sick or even die. In order to prevent any mishap they went to a mganga for medicines to prevent a new pregnancy and to protect their baby from illness.

This "birth control" medicine was not taken internally but consisted of a baobab rope treated with a type of medicine which the mganga would not reveal. Seven knots were tied in the rope which was then worn around the thigh of the woman. The informant added: "This is a very powerful pregnancy prevention. The mother will never catch pregnancy unless she unties the rope." Also, part of the treatment was to smear semen over the body of the baby to prevent sickness.

Nineteen waganga were asked specifically if people came to them for pregnancy prevention medicines, and all replied affirmatively. The interviews revealed that more clients seek medicine in order to conceive than for preventing pregnancies. Fifteen waganga specified that it was the men who came for help because they were impotent. No one had ever come for medicine to avoid having children completely, but rather for the aid of medicine in keeping the taboos necessary for protection of an unweaned child.

Because the Zaramo accept all children, whether in or out of wedlock, they do not generally consider the possibility of abortion. Again, of the 19 waganga who were approached on the subject of abortion, five admitted to knowing a medicine for abortion but only one admitted to having administered it. Almost all others considered abortion morally wrong, one calling it a "sin". Only very rarely do women ask a mganga for abortion medicine and indications are strong that in most instances the mganga would not comply. In this respect the traditional medicine man is a upholder of the generally accepted Zaramo moral code concerning abortion, killing or *uchawi*.

Others who were interviewed regarding the help they had received from waganga for sexual problems related the use of several medicines called *fungalunda*, *mbwa*, *fungakuni*, *kutega* and *usinga*. It was explained that these medicines could cause an adulterous husband or wife to become affixed to the other lover during the act of intercourse. In such an event only the legal marriage partner could release the lovers from each other, who would inevitably expose their unlawful act when calling for help. Whether or not such medicines are widely used or are even effective can be debated, but nevertheless every person questioned on the subject had knowledge of the medicines and several were able and willing to explain how they were made and used.

Five other informants described medicines and methods employed by wives to render their husbands impotent as punishment for unfaithfulness. With these treatments, as well as with the other allegedly effective medicines, the threat may be used only to create fear, thus putting a check on the actions of the suspected marriage partner. Impotency and barrenness are of much importance to the Zaramo, so it may be that these powers of punishment claimed by the waganga in fact act as sanctions in Zaramo society.

8. Sports

In the Zaramo war against the Kamba, thought to be around 1800, the leader, Pazi Kilama, employed waganga to make medicine with which to treat the warriors as well as the spears and arrows, so as to assure victory. In the 1905 Maji Maji rebellion, also, the participating Zaramo were treated with magical water to ward off bullets. Today the Zaramo are involved in no wars, but the waganga have adapted similar methods for protecting football players and winning their matches. This is the only area in this study where *uchawi*, as used against the opposite football team, was considered justifiable and proper.

The practice of consulting waganga for treatment of football players and for bewitching the opposing team is sufficiently common to have been mentioned by six out of sixty waganga as one of the problems referred to them. Four other waganga mentioned it as a problem rarely encountered. If the problem had appeared more often in the study one would have doubted the statistics because there are not enough football clubs in Dar es Salaam to provide all the waganga with business.

The following information has been derived from interviews with six football players from Dar es Salaam's two largest and most popular football clubs. Another player from a lesser known club supplied additional information, as did two football fans.

Mr. O.S., the secretary of one team, remarked, "Not some, but nearly all teams use much money on *uchawi*. It is very hard to escape it because nearly everyone on the team believes in it and will be afraid to play a game if they are not treated beforehand. So the leaders must employ waganga who know the medicine. A week before a football match the players must go to the appointed mganga to be treated. The waganga also come to treat the club premises so that the players will not be bewitched there. We must treat our best players so they do not break their legs or lose their strength. Sometimes a mganga is paid a thousand shillings for his services." He added: "The famous teams of Dar es Salaam do not agree to play football frequently, because the waganga's fees are so costly."

Football player C.B. described how he had medicine applied before a game. He said: "We went first to one mganga to get *dawa* for use in a bath in order to make the body strong. At a second mganga we got *dawa* with which to wash our legs. This was to protect the legs from *uchawi* used by the other team. We each were given a small red *hirizi*, amulet, to carry in our pockets during the match. After the game we had to return the amulets to the team manager. Our team leaders will not allow the team to play unless they have made *uchawi* against the other team."

Mr. J.C., another player, confided that he is afraid to play in big games because of the witchcraft used by the opposing teams. He fears getting his legs broken and thinks that if he becomes a popular player *uchawi* will be used against him more readily.

Player S.Y. stated: "The name of the team mganga must be kept secret. If not, the opposing team might pay him more money to give us weak medicine."

Two members of another team gave similar information. They disclosed that it is also common practice to consult a diviner to see who will win the match. If the diviner reveals that the team will be defeated on a particular day, they might refuse to play. This happened so frequently in 1967 and 1968 that the sports association was compelled to impose a fine of 1,000 shillings on any team which failed to appear for a scheduled match. In June 1967 the Cosmos Club was fined this amount when their team neglected to turn up for a game. And for six months the Sunderland team refused to play against the Young Africans because the omens were said to be against their winning.

Player K.M. related the following account of a football match held in Tanga in 1967. The opposing team was wearing black arm-bands because, they said, one of their team-mates had recently died. They offered black arm-bands to K.M.'s team, requesting the team to wear them out of respect for the deceased. In the course of the game K.M.'s team noticed that they were not as strong as usual and began to suspect the arm-bands. During the next quarter of the game they removed their arm-bands and immediately regained their strength, going on to win the game. Player K.M. commented with certainty: "They gave us the cloths to make us weak. There was medicine in the cloths."

Other informants said that the waganga sometimes applied medicine directly to the football field. They might even bury a chicken in the field during the night before a match, or they might secretly treat the ball or the hands of the players as a means of passing the *uchawi* on to the opponents. All these stories are the source of endless discussion and joking. The seriousness with which both players and waganga spoke of this work, however, indicates that for them it is no joking matter. Just as Pazi Kilama and the participants in the Maji Maji rebellion took no chances, so today the football teams in Dar es Salaam employ waganga for the same purpose.

A cartoon appearing in the April 22nd., 1968 issue of the Dar es Salaam Swahili newspaper *Ngurumo* illustrates both the humor and the seriousness of belief in the power of *uchawi* over football teams. The cartoon depicts a policeman watching a football player in uniform climbing up a ladder to pass over the wall surrounding the football field. The policeman calls to him: "Eee. . . you Pepe! (nickname for empty husk of grain). What are you doing? Is that the door for entering the football field?" The player replies: "No, sir it isn't. . . I fear to pass through the gate because they (the other team) have planted *uchawi* and if I go in there I might sprout into dates."

9. Politics

Only two waganga reported treatment of cases related to political affairs. No cases, however, appeared in their previous day's case loads nor did any appear amongst the 100 cases studied. Therefore I found no evidence for believing that Tanzanian politicians consult waganga about political affairs as is reported about some politicians in the West African states. It could be that the Zaramo politicians, as well as others, buy good luck medicines during election times, but this is based only on hearsay. No one could give me an eye-witness account. Even the rumors are related only to winning elections, seeking protection from sorcery, and seeking medicine to enhance popularity or to protect a political post.

One prominent NUTA secretary in Dar es Salaam commented: "Many of the politicians go to waganga for *dawa ya bahati*, medicine of luck. They have special waganga whom they contact before giving a speech, especially at public meetings. Walking sticks and whisks are treated with medicine. There are some special places where they go for this treatment, mainly to Tanga, but sometimes to Mlingotini." (Mlingotini is a coastal Zaramo village near Bagamoyo noted for its powerful waganga. Its name was often mentioned in interviews in connection with sorcery.)

Another informant explained how politicians have the ground and platform treated before election speeches in order to ensure popularity and to bewitch the opponent. This informant advises that the Bondei (from the Tanga Region) and the Zigua are particularly adept at making such medicines.

From the limited historical material available on the Zaramo I found no accounts of waganga entering community politics in the past. Today, however, a mganga might be elected as a TANU secretary or ten-house cell leader, but this would be on the basis of his leadership and popularity and not on his uganga skills. Muslim *shehe* and *mwalimu* have been active in coastal politics and several have been elected to political posts. They generally use their Muslim titles, but I have never noted anyone in politics or public affairs who had used the title "mganga". The Dar es Salaam waganga have assumed many roles in Zaramo society, but the political role is not one of them.

10. Miscellaneous: Good Luck, School Exams and Fortune Telling

A few waganga, in discussing their cases, referred to some clients as good luck seekers. It was explained that such people are looking for an amulet to help them pass a school examination, an exam for a particular job, or to help them win a lottery draw. One informant who had taken an examination for employment with the office of the National Treasury said that six other men who sat with him for the examination all carried amulets.

Four Zaramo students studying in Dar es Salaam secondary schools acknowledged that it is common practice for Zaramo students to by *dawa* from waganga or Muslim practitioners in order to pass examinations. Typical of their statements were those of S.M., a 16 -year - old schoolboy living in Kariakoo: "Medicines for exams are very helpful. It is better to help yourself with medicines before sitting for an exam. Medicines will help you especially on the correction day. The person who corrects your paper will just put good marks on your paper. His mind will be blinded and he won't see the mistakes. It is very good to study, but also much better to have medicines to help you at an examination time. Many have passed through this way, but you have to get a mganga who knows the medicine. Not every mganga knows. A *shehe* may read the Koran over you and give you a *hirizi*. Sometimes this helps very much, if that *shehe* knows his Koran well."

Three Zaramo Christian girls also confirmed this as a common practice. But at the same time they ridiculed the idea as foolish.

Fortune-telling is an apparently recent innovation popularized by Sheikh Yaka Hussein of Magomeni. He has published several astrology and horoscope books and his sensational predictions are invariably made known in the newspapers. Typical of his medical advice is that which he advertised in the Dar es Salaam *Nationalist* newspaper on April 22nd., 1968:

SOLVE YOUR PROBLEMS THIS WAY IN THE MONTH OF APRIL
- DOCTORS AND PATIENTS -

> During this month doctors are advised to inject, vaccinate or operate their patients on their right side.
>
> Telephone first to get your appointment with an astrologer. Stars forecast your future better than any kind of magic.

Sheikh Hussein may prefer to classify himself as an astrologer rather than a mganga, but his knowledge and function are similar to that of other *shehe* in the city. The only exception is that he has moved into the fortune-telling and horoscope business and understands modern techniques. He declined to answer any questions when interviewed. His political record and relationship to the East African Muslim organizations are interesting but have no specific relevance to the subject of this study.

Again we see in the brief illustrations of this last section how waganga have related themselves to present-day situations. They have adapted their skills and knowledge to meet the difficulties of the modern student. The waganga may not themselves be able to pass the exams or to secure better employment, but they are prepared to enable others to do so. In a time of rapid social change, when Zaramo as well as other people are confronted with new situations, increased tensions and an uncertain future in the urban world, the mganga offers good luck, fortune telling and confidence by administering the old and tried traditional medicines.

I have tried in this chapter to let the evidence in the client cases and the activity of the waganga speak for themselves. We have noted the various roles the mganga plays in his work connected with uganga. As a healer, protector, judge, success maker and diviner, he is firmly established in urban Zaramo life. By attributing the cause of illness and misfortune to sorcery, witches, broken taboos, ancestor spirits and spirit possession, we have seen that *the mganga continues to function as a preserver of traditional Zaramo social and religious patterns.*

The cases also revealed problems of jealousy due to material wealth, position, childlessness and marital relations. Underlying this jealousy are socio-economic factors caused by the insecurity of urban life and work, crowded housing conditions, inter-tribal suspicion, lack of education, and economic inequality. It was seen in the cases that *the new urban social environment, with its accompanying tensions, allows a new set of accusations to be proposed as an explanation for the cause of illness and misfortune*. This was seen most particularly in the increase in sorcery accusations as compared with rural accusations where spirits were thought to be the main cause.

The cases give evidence that the mganga is attempting to adapt his service to the modern urban needs of his clientele. The job seeker and the student before an examination receive good luck charms for success, the shopkeeper receives protection for his business, the football player is protected from his opponent, the suspicious husband or wife is given medicine to ward off new lovers, and the fear of sorcery by neighbors is relived. These new urban situations are treated with medicine and methods conforming to the Zaramo traditional understanding of life and spirit powers. The types of problems treated in these 100 client cases, and as revealed in the day's case load of 60 waganga, verify the hypothesis presented in this study, that *the mganga, a key person in preserving traditional Zaramo culture, continues to function in modern urban society by adapting his role to the changing social conditions of his clientele.*

Notes to Chapter 4

1)Chinduti K.Chirwa, "Post Mortem on Those Hospital Complaints: interview with Dr. A.D. Chiduo", *The Standard* (Dar es Salaam) September 1971.

2)Cases in each Table are numbered consecutively. The second number given ie. S.1, S.2 etc. refers to the number given to the case in the researcher's field notes.

3)Prince, Raymond, "Indigenous Yoruba Psychiatry" Ari Kiev, op. cit., p. 116.

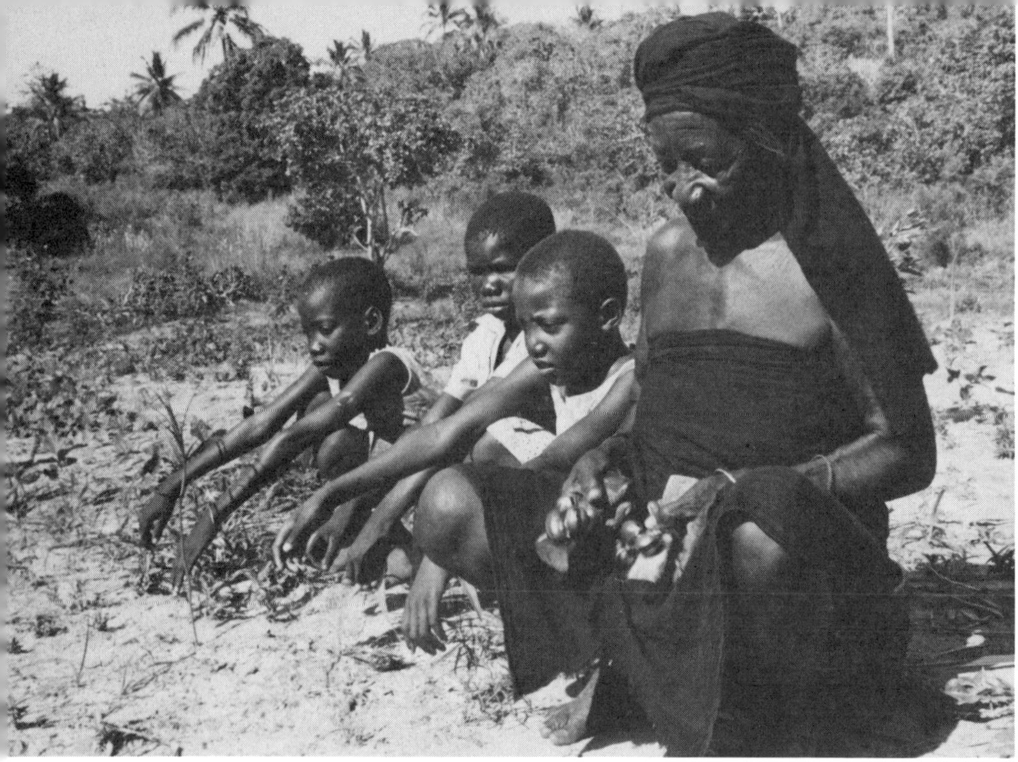

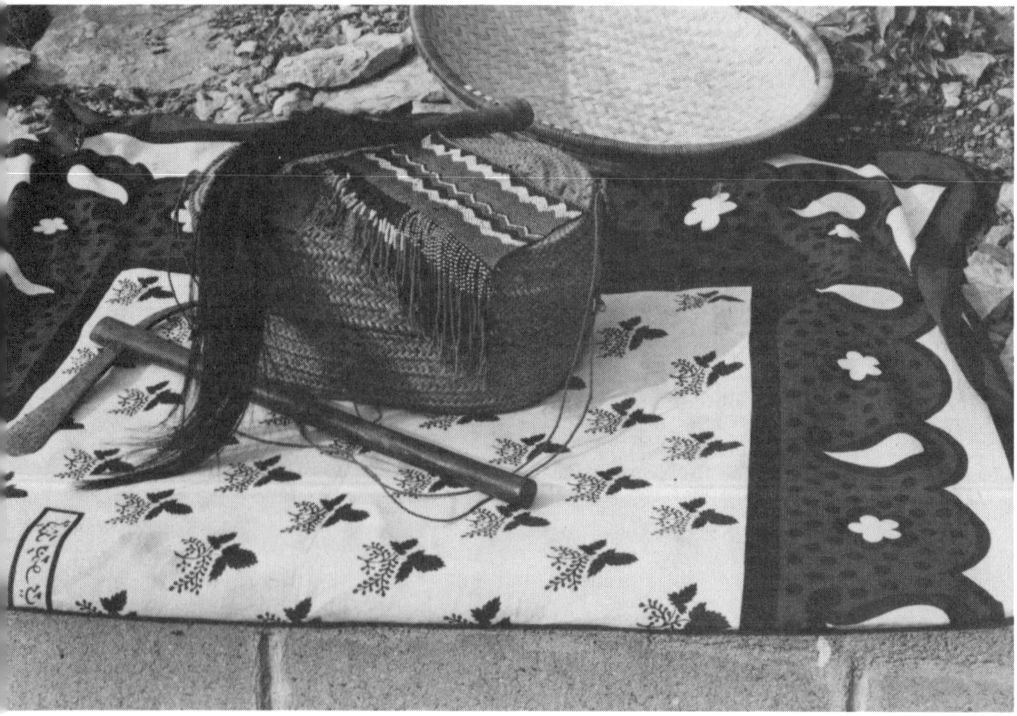

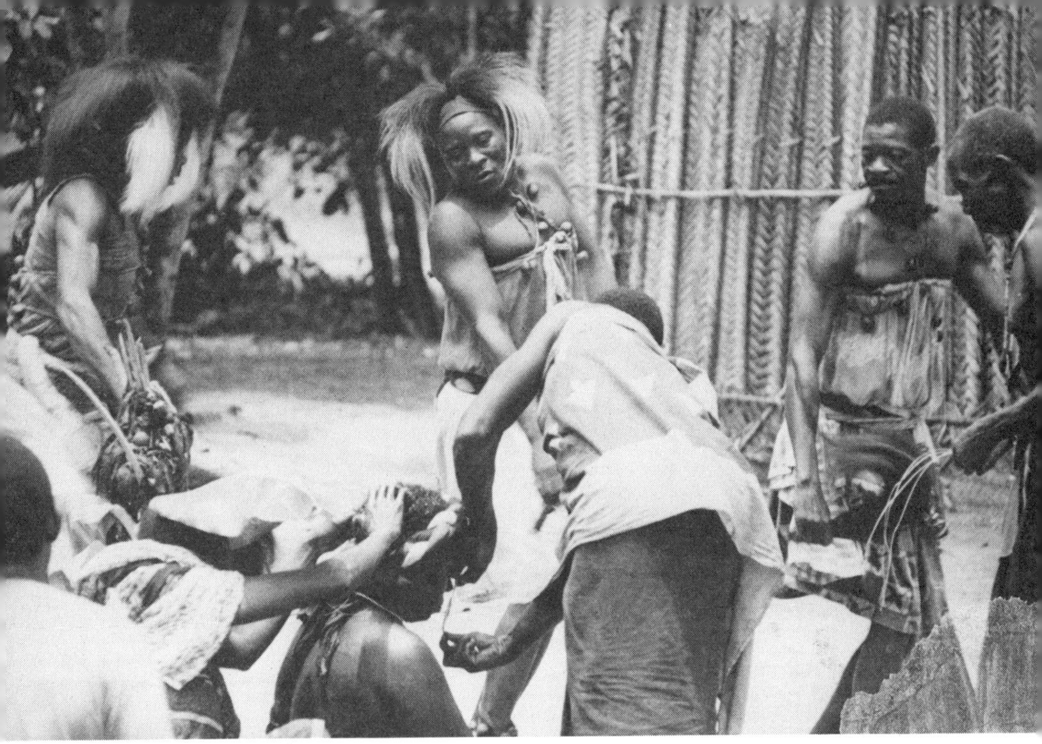

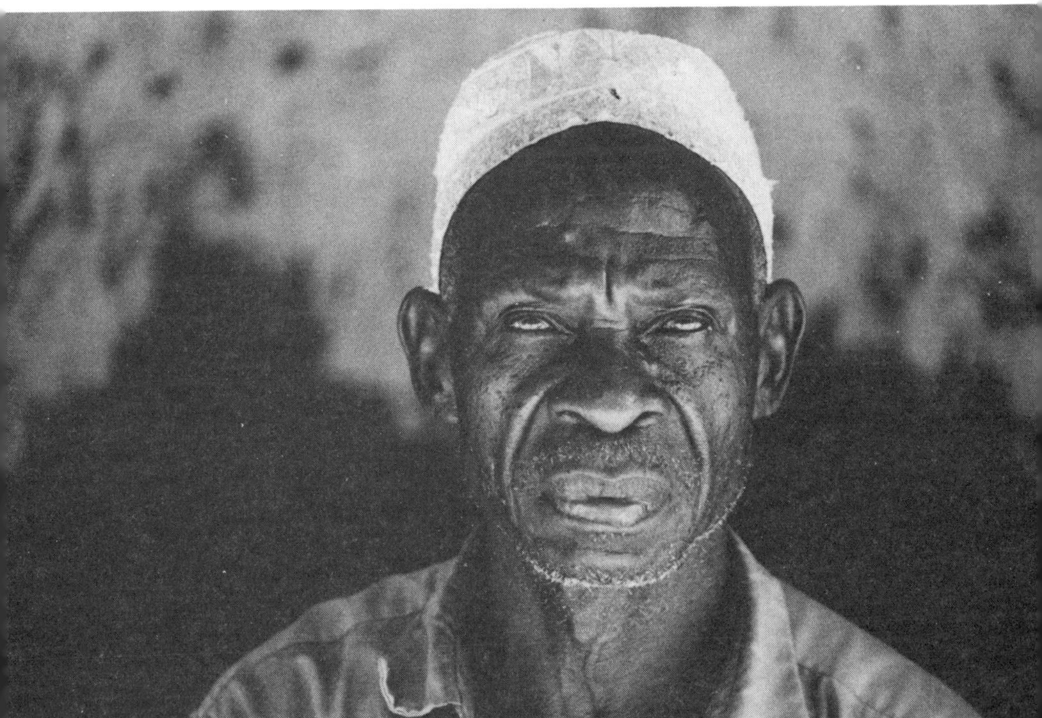

EXPLANATIONS TO THE PICTURES ON PAGES 132–133

P. 132 top: Mwawila, a Rungu spirit diviner and medicine woman, with her three little assistants, using the *kukiga ramli* method.

P. 132 bottom: Typical Zaramo medicine bag with the healer's symbols of office: an axe and a wild-beast tail whisk.

P.133 top: A Zaramo spirit exorcism — *Madagoli* with the client seated in the middle and three medicinemen dancing. Photo by Ingmar Lindqvist.

P. 133 bottom: A Kinyamhera spirit *mganga*, Sahron Hunzi. Photo by Ingmar Lindqvist.

CHAPTER 5
The Changing Role of the Medicine Man in Urban Zaramo Society

From the preceding material we have seen how at times it is Zaramo society, with its cultural beliefs and practices, which shapes the work of the mganga, while at the same time the mganga is shaping Zaramo thought and practice by the multiplicity of roles he plays in urban society. As urbanization has brought on change in the life style of the Zaramo and put them into new circumstances, so the mganga has adapted his practice to fit the needs of this urban situation.

The structural changes the Zaramo society has gone through in becoming urbanized are reflected in the changing concepts and practices concerning illness and misfortune. In this changing urban society the mganga emerges in a fairly strong position. He continues as a preserver of traditional Zaramo social and religious patterns and because of his apparent success he has maintained for himself a role in urban society. The mganga's role is not a static one but adapts itself to the new social situation and the needs of his clientele. He functions in a number of roles. Satisfactory performance of these roles legitimates his practice and offers a significant reason why this is not waning in urban society.

A summary of findings and further analysis of the points briefly outlined above are now given, and leads to the concluding statements about the success of the mganga in preserving his role in urban society. We turn first to the mganga amidst the structural changes in urban society.

1. The Consequences of Structural Change in Urban Zaramo Society

a. *Changing Accusations in a New Urban Environment:*

Earlier studies have given evidence that witchcraft and sorcery accusations are generally made against people within the kin-group. Tensions in rural societies developed between members of the kin-group who were in a competing position in one way or another. Tensions arose over title to land, competition for leadership and in some ethnic groups between father and son for wives. The most common assumption about such a competitor who was thought to be the cause of some illness or misfortune was that he or she was a witch.

The structural position of urban people is changing. They move in a new network of social relationships, acting in different roles in different spheres of life. Their urban conflicts have foci unknown in the rural context. Hence these changing relationships encourage new explanations for the causes of illness and misfortune.

The mganga/diviner is well aware of the tensions in urban Zaramo society caused by crowded housing conditions, inter-tribal jealousy and misunderstanding. The mganga knows the instability of the Zaramo marriage and the perpetual round of suspicions of infidelity between those living together in various forms of marriage. Leslie's social study, *A Survey of Dar es Salaam*, tells of the jealousies and hatred engendered over clothing, food, children and salaries, an account amply substantiated by the accusations reported in my 100-client case study.

Accusations against members of the kin-group were surprisingly few (only three) as compared with the numerous rural kin accusations. Because of the separation from rural kin while living in the city, the occasions for tensions are lessened. Tensions among kin over land, crops and trees are decreased because of the urban-rural separation. The Zaramo now sees his neighbor or his colleague, and not his kin members, as his competitor.

The diviner, not knowing the urban kin relationships, finds it easier and safer to focus blame for a problem on a neighbor. Only one of the three kin accusations recorded in the study involved inheritance of property. The other two instances were matters of jealousy over a higher position in a job and of misunderstanding in a marriage arrangement. In addition to this, two sorcery accusations were against husbands, one against a wife, and two against co-wives. Marital tensions resulting in accusations of sorcery seem to be about the same in intensity in both rural and urban situations, according to the statistics available.

Even when the spirits were blamed for a particular problem it may be noted that urban waganga avoided recommending exorcism as treatment. Five of the others were reprimanded for neglecting their ancestor graves and were given medicine as part of the treatment. They were further instructed to return to their home villages to make grave *tambiko* offerings. The other cases of spirit intervention were said to be such that they could be treated in the city with medicine and need not have exorcism. This proves very satisfactory for the client as well as the mganga, for it necessitates great trouble and expense to arrange a *madogoli* for which all the kin should be present.

The above illustrations from the study reveal how *the new urban situation allows the mganga to propose a new set of accusations as explanation of the cause of a problem and also how he adapts his treatment for convenience of the client as well as for his own financial benefit.*

b. *The Trend from Collective Support and Ritual Healing to Individual Responsibility and Healing :*

There is another factor in urban life which is related to the change in methods of curing. In the urban situation the pattern of social relationships differs from the rural pattern. There is a change in the intensity of kinship relations which result in lessening kinship support in cases of illness and misfortune. The urban Zaramo do not see their central problem within the context of the kinship group but rather their problems change in such a way as to reflect the importance of the new relationships. The Zaramo do not continue to look for solutions only within the kinship or tribal context.

Kin togetherness has always been considered one of the marks of traditional Zaramo society. People were never alone in their work or in their difficulties. All important events in their lives from birth to death were attended and supported by all members of their extended kin-group. They needed one another because life was often severe and fraught with danger from both human sources and those of the spirit world. Kin support was therefore necessary and could function effectively because the kin lived in the immediate vicinity. Treatment of disease and misfortune could be carried out with kin participation, and therefore such treatment was often recommended by waganga through divination. Spirit exorcism, the most common Zaramo rural treatment, is a method involving group therapy which requires the presence of the entire kinship group.

In Dar es Salaam the extended family situation is noticeably changing. Not all kin live in the city, and families are separated by distances which make communication between the rural and urban segments difficult. Urbanization therefore leads to reliance on the nuclear family and on individual responsibility. City workers cannot leave their jobs very often to attend a *madogoli* or the numerous rituals in the life cycle for which they should be present. Lack of money for travel often hinders the rural kin from visiting the city. Even to accommodate and feed the kin at such gatherings creates a problem, especially as extra urban housing is difficult to find.

In order to meet this urban situation the mganga shrewdly recommends a more convenient individual treatment of the problem rather than ordering group therapy which requires the presence of the extended family. This is more suitable to his client as well as to the mganga himself. Group rites generally take a day or two to perform, and a *rungu* may go on daily for weeks. In this same amount of time the mganga might more profitably treat 20 or 30 clients on an individual basis.

Kin togetherness and support is not altogether lacking in the city, but it is based more and more on the nuclear family members and not on the extended family. When a person is ill or has a problem it may be that he or she remains at home in bed while a family member goes to a diviner to find out who caused the trouble and what steps should be taken. It was discovered in the 58 divination sessions that 17 of the clients had remained at home while a member of the family went to a diviner on their behalf. All were members of the nuclear family. They were husband or wife, father or mother; none were cousins, uncles or just friends.

There are times when a member of the family will accompany a client to the mganga, especially in cases of mental illness. But a surprising number of clients make the visit alone.

In the 100 client cases no accusation was recorded as being made by one clan group against another. Accusers were individuals, never an entire family. It was noticeable that accusations were usually female against female and male against male.

Both the treatment and the counter-measure are seen as an individual responsibility. Because these are personal conflicts between individuals, often leading to revenge which they know to be wrong, people prefer to keep their problems a private matter. They understand that *uchawi* is contrary to the law and moral code of society, and they therefore avoid publicizing their problems lest they be accused of using sorcery for revenge.

Because of the new urban situation bringing separation to the extended family we have seen how individuals are placed in a position where they must handle their own problems without the help of others. At best they can rely on their nuclear family members for support in times of illness and misfortune.

We have seen in the case material one other changing aspect in the mganga's form of treatment. Marja-Liisa Swantz's study on *Ritual and Symbol* has revealed that much of the *uganga* in a rural society is directed toward ritual healing. Emphasis on social ritual has the effect of social healing. Not only is the individual exorcised from a troubling spirit but he or she must be surrounded by the kin-group. It is not only good group therapy for that individual, but family relationships can be cleared and kin and cult community can meet to affirm their togetherness. The healing situation is a social situation in which the social relationships are affirmed. By projecting the cause of the problem onto the spirits, the actual social relationships are not strained further. Through ritual action the social relationships are restored.

In the urban treatment of illness and misfortune we find very little ritual healing on a kin-group or community level. The *madogoli* exorcism rite, for example, is seldom performed in the city or recommended by urban waganga. The question was posed aş to whether the urban mganga's interpretation of illness and misfortune, and the methods he uses for curing, aim at healing social relationships or whether his role is in fact directed rather toward individual healing and solving individual problems. The latter seems to be the case, for out of 100 cases only seven times were methods of cure suggested which were in the nature of ritual healing, where the kin-group would normally be called in.

The case material in this study shows how the accusations of the person or factors contributing to the sorcery problems reflect the urban Zaramo's frustrations and fears. The diviner, knowing the insecurity and fears in Zaramo society, confirms and enlarges the tension by his diagnosis of the problem. The diviner sets out to eliminate the evil power. He directs the client to another mganga, or he himself sets out to project the client and punish the evildoer, who may not have existed in the first place. Clients return home satisfied that they have been released from the power of the enemy and assured that the culprits who attacked them have been severely dealt with and deterred from further malicious action.

From the material presented we can conclude that *there is a change from kinship support to individual responsibility, a change from the extended family and cult member support to individual and nuclear family support in the treatment of illness and misfortune.*

Although the urban mganga recognizes the social causes of the client's problems he does not take the approach of some Western psychiatrists who see their patients as part of a network of disturbed relationships. The mganga tends to increase the social conflict rather than to minimize it. He treats the individual patient psychologically in relation to other people but leaves the social group untouched.

2. The Role of the Medicine Man in Urban Dar es Salaam

The authority of the mganga's role has been questioned in this study. Who legitimates his authority for the various roles he has assumed? Just as the mganga upholds Zaramo tradition, so also the tradition upholds the mganga's position. It is a time-tested and respected profession. No one questions the rightness or wrongness of Zaramo *mila*, tradition. If born into it, it is quite unthinkable to change or to ignore one's *mila* and *jadi*. So also it would be quite unthinkable to question the role of the mganga and his right to exist in Zaramo society.

It is often assumed that increased education may undermine the mganga's position and that the educated youth will lose their respect for him. This has not happened to any appreciable degree among the Zaramo to date. Traditional medicine retains its place side by side with "scientific" Western medicine. The Zaramo believe each has its own place and use, depending on the nature of the problem to be treated.

The real test of the mganga's position is in his own ability and skill in treating troubled people. If his *uganga* is not effective, clients will not return to him or recommend him to others, eventually forcing him to go out of business. For the present, public opinion and demand assure the successful mganga a place in Zaramo urban society.

We have not seen any entirely new roles taken on by the medicine man in Dar es Salaam. For example, he has not entered into politics; he has not become a formal public religious leader trying to promote a revival in Zaramo traditional religion. The mganga has not tried to use Western medicines, nor has he pretended to possess the qualifications of a recognized government doctor.

On the basis of his case load and the problems presented by his clients, we can say that the mganga's role as healer, protector, arbitrator and success-maker remains essentially the same as it has been over the past 75 years. The only significant change is in his explanation of the causes of problems and in his methods of diagnosis and treating illness and misfortune. There are also new types of problems brought to him, resulting from the urban situation and new trends in modern living. But the mganga treats these problems with the same medicine that he has always used.

a. *The mganga as a preserver of traditional Zaramo social and religious patterns:*

The Zaramo mganga exists today as one of the sole surviving professional functionaries of traditional practices. As such he is symbolic link with the past. The Zaramo headman, *mndewa* or *Pazi*, has been replaced by the TANU executive officer and by the ten-house cell leader, but the mganga has been neither replaced nor outlawed by the Government or by modern medicine.

The mganga upholds the belief and practice of the ritual *tambiko* offering to ancestor spirits. He applies the sanctions against those who neglect both the ancestor spirit graves and other Zaramo traditional spirits. Urban Zaramo may become negligent in their ancestor obligations and therefore the mganga often advises them to make amends in fulfilling the *jadi*.

The mganga continues as an active medium between the Zaramo and their spirits. Although in the city he does not often exorcise the spirits

Kinyamkera, Mwenembago, Rungu or Ruhani, he may take his clients to the country to do so or refer them to other waganga of these spirits in the rural area. Far from denying the existence of the Zaramo spirit world, the waganga intensify belief in it and in the Zaramo ritual obligation by the word and treatment in their practice.

In promoting the exorcism rites the mganga is instrumental in strengthening Zaramo kin cohesion and in renewing the *ujamaa*, kin-togetherness, concept. The *madogoli* and *rungu* not only draw urban and rural kin together, but also stimulate community feeling among participants and spectators alike. Through exorcism rites the mganga indirectly promotes Zaramo traditional music, dance and mythology. Together with the life cycle rites, public exorcism and spirit rites are the strongest instruments for the advancement of Zaramo cohesion and consciousness.

Zaramo religion is not a set of doctrines but is rather the total Zaramo way of life - their thinking, believing and living. The Zaramo religion cannot be separated from the social, material and cultural aspects of their lives. It includes the natural order, the spiritual order as well as the *mila*, the traditional order. The mganga reinforces this Zaramo world-view by his own belief and medical practice, and in his counsel to others. No other public figure in Zaramo society today promotes and represents this "Zaramo-ness" of life in thought and action as does the mganga.

Aiding the mganga in strengthening Zaramo tradition is his continued use of the Zaramo language when singing traditional songs during the performance of the *madogoli*, *rungu* and *kilinge* rites as well as in *rungu* divining. It is the mganga who memorizes and passes on to others the chronology of waganga in the community and the names of all the spirits to be acknowledged in rituals and prayers. Where written accounts have never been made, it is in the oral traditions and rituals that Zaramo knowledge and beliefs are transmitted. The waganga are the public transmitters of the culture.

The mganga, perhaps more than any other person, preserves the knowledge of the names and uses of Zaramo herbs and medicines. As he trains an apprentice or one of his own kin to be a mganga, he is instrumental in transplanting Zaramo medical and botanical practices to the next generation.

The mganga helps to keep alive the knowledge and observance of clan taboos. From time to time he credits disease or calamity to the breaking of a taboo and arranges ritual cleansing accordingly. Without this occasional reminder the urban Zaramo would tend to forget the significance of clan taboos. Again this strengthens clan cohesion and consciousness.

As a leader of a kin-group or spirit cult group, the mganga does not function as effectively in urban Zaramo society as does his rural counterpart. Nevertheless he does return to the rural area from time to time to make his own ritual offering at the ancestor grave or spirit hut, and on such an occasion might assist in the prayers. It can be assumed, however, that to urban Zaramo he is a symbol of clan and cult unity even though within the city environment he is not a recognizable leader of such groups. On the other hand this study shows that the urban mganga does not operate along tribal lines; he treats all who come to him regardless of their tribe or religion. Likewise clients do not seek out a mganga of their own tribe, but rather go to the one with the best reputation. Waganga are willing to learn from those of another tribe, resulting in a general diffusion of *uganga* methods amongst coastal people. However, in the main we see in his practise that *the mganga continues to function as a preserver of traditional Zaramo social and religious patterns.*

b. *The Multiplicity of the Mganga's Roles:*

i. The Role of Healer

This study contains sample quantitative evidence to prove that the mganga is still well-established in his traditional role as a healer of illness. Some 700 waganga are engaged in this full-time business in Dar es Salaam and the number is likely to grow, not to diminish. The mganga himself claims healing to be his predominant activity. In the report of a single day's case load enlisting 60 medicine men, it has been noted that 338 clients were treated for various organic illnesses. Transferring this ratio to the estimated 700 waganga working in Dar es Salaam, it can be assumed that approximately 5,000 people are treated every day by medicine men for this cause alone.

The range of illnesses treated includes such a variety as stomach problems, dizziness, tuberculosis, mental illness, menstrual problems, heart, chest, body, leg and arm pains, pregnancy difficulties, fertility difficulties and snake-bites. The mganga willingly treats any type of illness and claims to know various combinations of medicine, both herbal and magical, which can cure the client. If his own *dawa* is not powerful enough he may refer the client to another mganga.

On some occasions the mganga may refer a client to a hospital, especially if he considers the problem to be a "European sickness". Sixteen per cent of the Zaramo clients interviewed had in fact first gone to a hospital for treatment but, discouraged by continued illness, transferred to a traditional medicine man. The numbers who have gone to a medicine man and then to the hospital because of his failure to cure them have not been measured in this study, but reports from doctors indicate that such cases are relatively common and often tragic. Deaths resulting from traditional medical treatment were on the increase in the 1960s, according to the Government Chemist.

We have no way of assessing the mganga's success in healing, other than to note that clients would not continue to seek him in such large numbers if they were not satisfied with his service. His knowledge of herbs, some of which have medically-acknowledged therapeutic properties, his interest in the client as a person, his understanding of the wholeness of people and his reliance upon the help of God, all contribute to his image within Zaramo society as a successful healer.

Zaramo healers, like the Yoruba, often do not make a clear distinction between physical disease and psychoneuroses. This may be so because Zaramo neurosis largely presents itself in physical symptoms.

Current psychiatric theory treats psychic diseases as expressions of disturbed relationships between people. Individuals are set in a network of relationships which affect them. When they become ill the causal interpretation may be sought within the organic sphere or within their situation in their social field.

The belief and fear of witchcraft and sorcery, together with the insecurity brought on by urban social change, may be an explanation for the large number of cases of illness coupled with sorcery accusations. If these illnesses treated by the medicine man are cured it may well be because the majority of the disorders were caused by psychological processes. The nature of the problem is such that the mganga has success in curing it with his traditional methods because these recognize the shaken social relationships as a causal factor and lean heavily on restoring security and peace of mind in the affected individual.

The Zaramo's concept of causes of illness and misfortune can be described as belonging to the same three categories that Raymond Prince recognizes in his study of the Yoruba: the natural, preternatural and supernatural. For the physical aspect the medicine man gives herbal treatment; for the preternatural, mainly sorcery, he carries out a magical act to counteract the sorcerer's power; to placate the supernatural, the client may be asked to make a ritual sacrifice or offering. One or all three procedures may be carried out to complete the cure, so that at least in one area the client may feel some sense of relief.

Apart from the clients' experience of relief, it is still questionable, however, if the waganga have successfully handled their clients' psychoneuroses simply by giving them security through magical protective medicine. The shaken social relationships would need to be faced through some form of reconciliation. More likely the act of sorcery was not real in the first place, but imagined by the client or accepted as fact through the suggestion of the mganga. The mganga, instead of minimizing or healing social tensions, perpetuates social mistrust, giving only temporary satisfaction until a similar situation brings on another cycle of fear, and physical and psychological illness.

ii. The Role of Diviner

In the diagnosis of illness and misfortune the medicine man's role as a diviner continues as in the past. Approximately 80 per cent of Dar es Salaam waganga practice divining. All Muslim *shehe* and Koranic teachers stated that they divine and are in fact considered the most skilled at it. The Islamic forms of geomancy divining are used by waganga more than any other method. The traditional Zaramo forms of divining, such as that of *bao* and *rungu*, are used by only half of the waganga in the city today. This change is attributed to the influence of Islam and its more sophisticated methods of divining.

Of the 100 clients, 58 per cent had first gone for *ramli*, divining, to determine the cause of their problems. Others suffered types of illness or misfortune which readily revealed to them the cause; thus there was no need for a diviner's skill. With well over half of the clients, numbering approximately 2,000 to 3,000 per day, going for divination, it is clearly seen that the role of the diviner remains well-established and accepted. The mganga's role as diviner, seer, prophet, the one who knows the secrets of people and society, puts him in a class of his own. He or she is a person of mystery, possessing secret powers, a person to be respected and sought after in times of difficulty and uncertainty. That he or she has the answers is accepted without question by the client. The mganga in the role of diviner has the authority and position to function as a preserver of traditional Zaramo social and religious patterns.

In the urban society the role of the mganga, particularly in his capacity as a diviner, has also a socially divisive aspect. The mganga as a diviner makes the analysis of social causes and thus affects the social relationships. By suggesting sorcery as a cause, and pointing to definable persons as the guilty ones, it may be said that the mganga can momentarily alleviate the client's anxiety over his or her trouble, but at the same time he perpetuates and intensifies social mistrust in general.

iii. The Role of Protector

The mganga in the role of protector against the forces of evil, both human and spirit, has been well-established in rural traditional society and gives no indication of diminishing in urban Dar es Salaam. The fear of evil spirits, sorcerers and *jini* is very great and their presence is recognized by all Muslim Zaramo. As long as fear is present, the need for protection will continue.

Waganga consider the treatment of sorcery problems to be their second greatest activity. One hundred and fifty eight cases of sorcery were treated by 60 waganga in one day. In addition to this, 120 clients were given protective medicine against sorcery. Among the 100 client cases , 63 per cent were being treated because of the real or imagined work of sorcery. The extent of sorcery accusations and the accompanying fear which drives people to seek the medicine man's help is an index of the tensions existing in urban Zaramo society. This problem could well add up to some 3,500 to 4,000 sorcery cases being treated each day by waganga in Dar es Salaam.

Fear of witchcraft and sorcery has been listed by sociologists as one of the reasons for the movement of rural dwellers to the city. It has been my observation that sorcery accusations and fear of sorcery are two of the main reasons why Africans move so often to other areas within the city itself.

The mganga, by assuming the role of protector against sorcery, actually becomes the promoter of sorcery accusations and the accompanying tensions. Illness and the frustrations of urban life substantiate the belief that magical powers used in sorcery do exist, and the mganga's divination only confirms this suspicion, after which he offers his healing and protection against the sorcerer's power. All along, the general Zaramo public suspects that the "protector", be he mganga, *mwalimu* or *shehe*, is actually the same person who sells his powers to bewitch people. This is denied by most waganga, who look upon sorcery as an evil antisocial act. Who then, are the sorcerers? My contention is that they are largely, although not entirely, figments of the imagination, but very real in the minds of the people. Here again the mganga, through his offer of protection, alleviates the immediate fear but at the same time perpetuates the system of belief which is the underlying cause of the tension.

iv. The Judicial Role

To a small degree today the mganga has a judicial role in Zaramo society. He issues oaths and ordeals, thereby becoming a judge, arbitrator and a peacemaker among those who are willing to bring their problems to him. Married couples who suspect each other of illicit sex affairs come for ordeals to prove their innocence or to have an *Amini* oath read to assure each other by a curse of death that they will remain faithful. Ordeals may reveal the guilty, as well as clear people of thievery or sorcery charges. The account of mganga Nguvumali/Matoroka contained in the study indicates how popular and accepted is the work of witchcraft eradicators in present-day Dar es Salaam.

v. The Role of Success Maker

Finally we have seen the mganga in the hero-like role. When human resources fail to meet the tests and demands of urban society, the mganga emerges as a hero figure offering success to those who seek his help. For the weak and those who suffer failure and frustration, the mganga offers the way to succeed in urban life. Unemployment and the fear of losing a job in the urban situation are new experiences for many Zaramo. The mganga therefore provides medicine for those seeking work or in need of protecting a position of work. This appears to be one of his growing services. Success as well as protection for a store business, a market stall, prostitution or beer brewing can be assured by the mganga's magical medicine.

In the city where competition is intense and inter-personal relationships more complex, success in love-making and in attracting the opposite sex can be guaranteed with the *dawa* of the mganga. Likewise, such sensitive family problems as fertility, virility and birth control are considered "a very simple matter" by all medicine men interviewed on the subject. The mganga's self-assurance in this field must give much relief to people plagued with sexual problems. Fear of barrenness and impotency ranked high in the waganga's case load and was one of the main areas of conflict in both monogamous and polygamous households.

This study has given evidence also to the mganga's hero role in helping football teams and players wishing to win a match, or in influencing legal cases or examination results at school. The medicine men claim power to win elections, to shorten prison terms or to win a court case. In all of these we see the mganga adapting his skills to help Zaramo in new urban situations. In the past he used his powers to win wars; today he helps to win football matches or a lover. Where a person is not equal to the new tests of society, the mganga offers aid. His *dawa* gives confidence of success, encouragement in approaching a new girl or a potential employer, and sometimes success is in fact realized. Whether the medicine itself has any positive effect is yet to be tested, but it may indeed be a great psychological aid to the client.

On the other hand, we might ask if the mganga really succeeds in helping the client. Might students be deceived into thinking they will pass their examinations with the aid of a good luck charm rather than through the process of hard study? Might people become blind to their own poor working habits and failures in relationships by thinking that a good job can be secured or an election won with an amulet and a little *dawa* ? The underlying social problems remain untouched by the mganga. The shortage of jobs, the lack of occupational training, or economic instability may be the source of unemployment. Neither the mganga's medicine nor his sphere of influence touches these problems. Crowded housing conditions, ease in obtaining a divorce, and the breakdown of controls in urban society are some of the factors contributing to accusations of sorcery. These ills cannot be treated with medicine but must be considered on another level, a political and social level, for which the mganga has no authority nor apparent concern.

I do not believe the waganga are charlatans, but I do believe they deceive themselves and their clients by not being able to face up to the real problems of life. Their medicine may offer comfort or instill temporary confidence, but also blinds the recipient to the underlying medical, educational and socio-economic problems which remain unsolved.

3. Conclusions: The Mganga and Modern Medical Service

The relationship of the mganga to modern medical services is an area of great interest but is not covered by documentation in this study. To reject the traditional waganga outright is to deny ourselves the benefit of any possible contribution by them to human welfare. If we accept their work *in toto* and recommend it to the general public we may also do great disservice, for we will be accepting certain religious, magical and mythological beliefs and practices which are contrary to sound medical science and to the religious conscience of many.

The thinking public and the Ministry of Health cannot afford to ignore the presence of the traditional waganga who operate in such large numbers and who collect such vast sums of money from their clients. Even to study the financial aspect of traditional medical practice would be worthwhile for the tax-collectors. Traditional practitioners need no government grants or subsidies and they never complain about being underpaid !

We might also ask if today it is really objective or correct to write a history of medical services in Tanzania without including the age-old and continuing practice of the mganga. On the basis of the material in this study it is apparent that there needs to be a reappraisal of Tanzanian medical history for the sake of learning how illness and human difficulties were and are understood and treated by vast numbers of people in the country today.

It has been shown in the foregoing summary and analysis that *the mganga, a key person in preserving traditional Zaramo culture, continues to function in modern urban society by adapting his role to the changing social conditions of his clientele*. In the movement from rural to urban living, for thousands of Zaramo the mganga has been a symbolic figure, representing what was good in Zaramo tradition. The mganga is the bridge which helps the Zaramo adjust to the modern world. When the Zaramo cannot understand or endure the tests of modern society, the mganga offers that needed comfort and magical power to sustain them.

From the point of view of modern development the mganga is a traditionalist who perpetuates traditional concepts, yet he handles psychological and social problems which might otherwise lead to even worse personal and social conflicts. I suggest that the mganga practising in a more integrated rural society, with closer family and kin-relationships, directs more of his analysis of the problem and cure towards socially constructive methods which affirm social relationships, whereas the urban mganga's treatment is more individualistic and socially divisive.

The mganga, however, performs his services in the spirit of helpfulness; he does not force himself onto anyone. All may avail themselves of the help he has to offer and are free to walk away if they do not believe or trust his advice. Many educated and Christian Zaramo accept the mganga's herbal treatments, but depending upon the strength of their own beliefs, have little to do with his magic. For many others the mganga's view of illness, encompassing the organic, psychic, spiritual and social aspects of life as a whole, is thought to be closer to the truth than that of a medical practitioner who sees only organic disorder as the cause of illness. The mganga's understanding of psychosomatic illness might indeed be a more accurate assessment of the nature of illness than that of the dominant approach in modern medicine which separates the psychic from the physical and prescribes medicine for the latter only. Theories in modern medical practice are changing, however, and therapeutic centers have been established involving teams of medical doctors, psychiatrists, clergymen and social welfare workers. Such experiments have shown surprisingly positive results. The traditional waganga have perhaps unknowingly incorporated several of these professions into their own one-person system. Their practice has some valuable insights to give to the rational medical practitioners of today. Without a doubt their overall medical skills have secured for them a place in urban society and the Zaramo will not soon abstain from seeking their services.

My intention has not been to glorify or idealize the Zaramo past with its varied and rich tradition, nor to either glorify or dispute the role of the mganga in it. My effort has been primarily an attempt to describe and analyze. Those who live in Zaramo society may better judge the values and disadvantages of traditional medicine. The Zaramo are an important people but little understood in the nation's capital. In understanding them, and helping them to move forward to a better and healthier life, this city and nation will also enjoy a better and healthier life.

In what was intended to be an urban social change study of the Zaramo, the traditional mganga emerged as the most important public figure in the cultural life of the average Zaramo. His varied roles tell us much about the life and problems of both rural and urban Zaramo today. What remains to be seen is whether Tanzanian society as a whole can capture the dynamic forces in this traditional institution and utilize them for the development and good of the total community.

GLOSSARY

-agua	Sw.	to divine; foretell; *uagazi*, divination; *mwaguzi*, a diviner. More commonly spoken of by the Zaramo today as *kutazamia* or *kupiga ramli* or *bao*, to divine.
bao	Sw.	a board; an African game: In the context of this study it is the term used to describe a type of divination, *kupiga bao* (see *ramli*) often using a board, but sometimes sand on the ground, onto which objects are thrown.
dawa	Sw.	medicine; the name applied to almost any medicament given by a medicine man, including amulets and magical charms. The two main types are *dawa za miti* or *shamba*, herbal medicines, and *dawa ya kitabu*, medicines or treatments made with the Koran or other Islamic books.
dini	Sw.	religion, creed. The *dini* of the traditional Zaramo may be termed as *Upazi* or *Kipazi*.
halubadili	Sw.	(Ar. *Hal Badiri*, *Ahl al-Badr*) a curse, oath or liturgical incantation which is read when there is reason to suspect someone of an evil deed. It is also a form of an ordeal which may clear one of a sorcery accusation. This incantation incorporates portions of Koranic passages dealing with the battle of Badr and lists the names of warriors which helped to gain the victory.
hirizi	Sw.	(Ar. *hirz*) a charm or amulet to ward off evil. Also can be worn or carried when taking exams or seeking work. Also called a *kinga*, Sw.
jadi	Sw.	an ancestral or traditional obligation. Can also mean lineage, ancestor, genealogy, or origin.
jando	Sw.	the Swahili-Islamic name given to circumcision and initiation rite was known as *kula* or *nghula*, Z.
jini	Sw.	pl. *majini* (Ar. *djinn*) a spirit; usually applied to coastal spirits which are considered dangerous and often bloodthirsty.
kinga	Sw.	a protection amulet to ward off evil.

Kinyamkera	Sw.	a Zaramo female spirit around which a spirit possession cult has grown.
kipazi	Sw.	used in this study as the term covering Zaramo traditional beliefs and customs; Lit. the things of Pazi kilama, the alleged father of the Zaramo ethnic group. *Upazi* as a collective noun also has the meaning of Zaramo traditions, beliefs and customs.
kitabu	Sw.	a book; but meaning in the context of this study the Koran or other Islamic writings. *Dawa ya kitabu* refers to medicine or therapy through the means of Islamic writings.
Kolelo	Z., Lu.	a spirit shrine located in the Uluguru Mountains, visited by Luguru, Zaramo, Zigua and others. A spirit associated with a snake.
kungu	Sw.	pl. *makungu*, an ancestor spirit.
madogoli	Sw., Z.	a Zaramo spirit possession cult connected with Kinyamkera and Mwenembago spirits; the exorcism rite itself; sometimes refers to the dance connected with the rite. The name is the plural form of the *dogoli* drum played during exorcism rites.
mchawi	Sw.	pl. *wachawi*, a sorcerer; a wizard; one who practices so-called black magic. A witch may sometimes be called an *mchawi*, but in this study, unless specified, it refers to a sorcerer. See definitions in the text. *Uchawi*, witchcraft, sorcery, black magic.
mfuko	Sw.	bag, pocket; in this study the *mfuko* refers to a medicine man's bag where he keeps his medicine containers.
mganga	Sw.	pl. *waganga*, a medicine man or woman; doctor; in this study *mganga* refers to the traditional medical practitioner, while doctor refers to a scientifically trained doctor. A *mganga* can be diviner as well as a healer. The Zaramo language uses the same word as in Swahili. *Uganga*, the practice of medicine; the art of healing; can also mean medicine or amulets.
mila	Sw.	tradition, custom, habit.

mteja	Sw.	pl. *wateja*, the client or person who is being treated and exorcised by a mganga; also one who has been exorcised and now belongs to the spirit cult.
mumiani	Sw.	a dark-colored gum-like substance used by some Arabs and Asian as medicine; coastal people think it is coagulated blood taken from murdered victims, hence *mumiani* refers to people who are thought to murder people to steal their blood.
mwali	Sw.	a girl or a boy before or while in the initiation period. Often refers to Zaramo girl initiant in seclusion.
mwalimu	Sw.	pl. *walimu*, a teacher; a Muslim teacher or clerk; it refers in this study mainly to Muslim Koran teachers and some medicine men who have accepted the title, but have never taught or are no longer teaching or practising Muslim clerics.
mwanga	Sw.	pl. *wanga*, a witch, one who walks or flies in the night.
mwaguzi	Sw.	a diviner; see *-agua*. Usually a women in Zaramo society, but not necessarily so.
muwizi	Sw.	a circumciser.
ngoma	Sw.	a drum; a dance; in the Zaramo and East African context it denotes the total performance or ritual in which drums are used. *Ngoma* can also be translated as ritual, depending on the context in which it is used.
Pazi		a Zaramo clan name; often the title used to designate a village or area headman, *mndewa* Z. *Pazi kilama*, the early Kutu leader and "father" of those who call themselves Zaramo. From this name has originated the clan, the title, and also *kipazi* and *upazi* which designate traditional religion and custom. (See *kipazi*). P in Zaramo has developed from nasal mh; the title for a headman was earlier *mhazi*.
ramli	Sw.	(Ar. *Ramal*) also *uramli*, *uaguzi* and *ubashiri*, Sw., divination; *mpiga ramli*, a diviner; sometimes *mwaguzi*, Sw., diviner (See *-agua*).
rungu	Lu.	pl. *marungu* Sw., a snake spirit; an exorcism rite; a type of spirit divining with the use of ball-rattles. (See text)

shehe	Sw.	pl. *washehe* (Ar. *shaikh*), a sheikh, a leader in the Muslim religious order; a scholar in traditional Islamic law; an elder. The term is used very loosely in Zaramo and Swahili society. Often it is used interchangeably with *mwalimu.*
shetani	Sw.	pl. *mashetani* (Ar. shaytan), applied to a spirit of any description but more often to evil spirits which affect people. The word can mean Satan, but in Zaramo Muslim society *ibilisi* corresponds more to the English word devil or Satan. *Zezeta*, pl. *mizezeta*, Z., is the older expression for the *shetani* type of spirits, but is seldom used today.
tambiko	Sw.	usually translated as offering or sacrifice, usually connected with ancestor or other spirits at a grave or spirit hut.
uchawi	Sw.	sorcery; the practice of sorcery generally, whether by a sorcerer, *mchawi*, or by a *mganga.*
uganga	Sw.	medicine; the practice of medicine. In this study it refers to the practice of traditional medicine.
ukoo	Sw.	*lukolo*, Z., clan, kinship, descent, lineage. In the case of matrilineal Zaramo the biological descent follows the line of mother; certain ritual observances follow the *ukoo* of the father, which is called *mtala*, Z.
upazi		See *Pazi*, *kipazi.*
utani	Sw.	joking relationship; familiar friendship. *mtani*, pl. *watani*, those who practise *utani*, often in the form of abuse, jesting or burial obligations.

BIBLIOGRAPHY

Books

Beattie, John and Middleton, John (ed.) *Spirit Mediumship and Society in Africa.* London: Routledge and Kegan Paul, 1969.

Beidelman, T.O. *The Matrilineal Peoples of Eastern Tanzania.* London: International African Institute, 1967.

Carothers , J.C. *The African Mind in Health and Disease. A Study in Ethnopsychiatry.* World Health Organization, Monograph series No. 17. Geneva, 1953.

Davy, J.B. (ed.) *Check-List of Forest Trees and Shrubs of the British Empire, No. 5 Tanganyika Territory,* Part I. Oxford: Imperial Forestry Institute, 1940.

Douglas, Mary. "Techniques of Sorcery Control", *Witchcraft and Sorcery in East Africa.* Ed. by Middleton, J. and Winter, E.H. London: Routledge and Kegan Paul, 1963.

Douglas, Mary. *Witchcraft, Confessions and Accusations.* London: Tavistock Publications, 1970.

Evans-Pritchard, E.E. *Witchcraft, Oracles and Magic Among the Azande.* Oxford: Clarendon Press, 1937.

Field, M.J. *Search for Security.* London: Faber and Faber, 1962.

Fortes, M. and Dieterlen, G. (ed.) *African Systems of Thought.* London: International African Institute, Oxford University Press, 1965.

Garlick, Phyllis L. *Man's Search for Health. A Study in the Inter-Relation of Religion and Medicine.* London: The Highway Press, 1952.

Gelfand, Michael. *Witchdoctor, Traditional Medicine Man in Rhodesia.* London: Harvill Press, 1964.

Kiev, Ari. (ed.) *Magic, Faith and Healing. Studies in Primitive Psychiatry Today.* New York: Free Press, 1964.

Krelle, H. *Habari za Wazaramo.* Lushoto: Usambara Agentur, 1935.

Lambo, T. Adeoye, "Patterns of Psychiatric Care in Developing African Countries", in *Magic, Faith and Healing.* Ed. by Kiev, Ari. New York: Free Press, 1964.

Leighton, A.H., et. al., *Psychiatric Disorder Among the Yoruba.* Ithaca: Cornell University Press, 1963.

Leinhardt, Peter (ed.) *The Medicine Man, Swifa ya Nguvumali* (by Hasani bin Ismail). Oxford: The Oxford Library of African Literature, 1968.

Leslie, J.A. *A Survey of Dar es Salaam.* London: Oxford University Press, 1962.

Mair, L. *Witchcraft.* London: Weidenfeld and Nicolson, World University Library, 1969.

Marwick, M.G. *Sorcery in its Social Setting.* Manchester: Manchester University Press, 1965.

Marwick, M.G. (ed.) *Witchcraft and Sorcery.* Harmondsworth: Penguin Books Ltd. 1970.

Middleton, John (ed.) *Magic, Witchcraft and Curing.* American Museum Sourcebooks in Anthropology. New York: Natural History Press, 1967.

Midleton, John and Winter, E.H. (ed.) *Witchcraft and Sorcery in East Africa.* London: Routledge and Kegan Paul, 1963.

Mitchell, J.C. "The Meaning in Misfortune for Urban Africans" in *African Systems of Thought.* Ed. by Fortes, M. and Dieterlen, G. London: Oxford University Press, 1965.

Mwaruka, R. *Masimulizi Juu ya Uzaramo.* London: Macmillan, 1965.

Mzuanda, C. *History of Uluguru.*
Dar es Salaam: Privately published for Luguru Native Authority, 1958.

Orley, John H. *Culture and Mental Illness-A Study from Uganda.*
Nairobi: Publ. for Makerere Institute of Social Research, East African Publishing House, 1970.

Prince, Raymond. "Indigenous Yoruba Psychiatry",
in *Magic, Faith and Healing.* Ed. by Kiev, Ari.
New York: Free Press, 1964.

Siirila, Aarne. *The Voice of Illness.*
Philadelphia: Fortress Press, 1964.

Southall, Aidan. *Social Change in Modern Africa.* International African Seminar.
London: Oxford University Press, 1961.

Southall, A.W. and Gutkin, P.C.W. *Townsmen in the Making. Kampala and its Suburbs.* Kampala: East African Institute of Social Research.

Swantz, L.W. *The Zaramo of Tanzania.*
Dar es Salaam: Nordic Tanganyika Project, 1966.

Swantz, M-L. *The Religious and Magical Rites Connected with the Life Cycle of Women in Some Bantu Ethnic Groups in Tanzania.*
Dar es Salaam: Offset print of thesis manuscript, 1966.

Swantz, M-L. *Ritual and Symbol in Transitional Zaramo Society, with special reference to women.* Studia Missionalia Upsaliensia XVI.
Uppsala: Almqvist & Wiksells, 1970.

Swantz, M-L. *Zaramo Jando Rites in Mwambao Area.*
Research Reports No. 190.
Institute of Sociology, University of Helsinki, 1973.

Trimingham, Spencer J. *Islam in East Africa.*
Oxford: Clarendon Press, 1964.

Turner, V.W. *Schism and Continuity in an African Society.*
Manchester University Press for the Rhodes-Livingstone Institute, 1957.

Willis, R.G. "The Kamcape Movement".*Witchcraft and Sorcery.* Ed. by Marwick, M. London: Penguin Modern Sociology Readings, 1970.

Van Velsen, J. "The Extended-Case Method and Situational Analusis", *The Craft of Social Anthropology.* Ed. by Epstein, A.L. London: Tavistock Publications, 1967.

Articles and Periodicals

Baker, E.C. "Mumiani", *Tanganyika Notes and Records,* No. 11 (1941) 1-10.

Brown, Walter T. "Bagamoyo", *Tanzania Notes and Records,* No. 71 (1970) 83.

Chirwa, Chinduti K. "Post Mortem on Those Hospital Complaints: Interview with Dr. A.D. Chiduo", *The Standard,* Dar es Salaam (Sept. 1971) 4.

Cory, Hans. "Jando ya Zaramo", No. 165. Hans Cory Papers, Library, Dar es Salaam, University of Dar es Salaam.

Cory, Hans. "Notes on Zaramo Jando", File 109. Library, University of Dar es Salaam.

Cory, Hans. "Dar es Salaam, City Port and Region", *Tanzania Notes and Records,* No. 71. (Dar es Salaam, 1954).

Imperato, P.J. "Witchcraft and Traditional Medicine among the Luo of Tanzania", *Tanganyika Notes and Records,* No. 66 (Dar es Salaam, 1966) 193.

Johoda, G. "Traditional Healers and Other Institutions Concerned with Mental Illness in Ghana", *International Journal of Social Psychiatry,* Vol. 7 (1961) 245-268.

Klamroth, M. "Beiträge zum Verständnis der religiosen Vorstellungen der Saramo im Bezirk Dar es Salaam", *Zeitschrift für Kolonialsprachen.* Bd. I (Berlin,1910-1911) 37-72, 118.153, 189-223.

Klamroth, M. "Religionsgespräche mit einem Führer der Das es Salaamer Mohammedaner", *Allgemeine Missions-Zeitschrift*, V (1913) 65-80.

Koritschoner, Hans. "Details of a Native Medical Treatment", *Tanganyika Notes and Records*, No. 2 (1936) 67-71.

Krauss, Hans. "Volksmedizinische Beobachtungen bei den Küstennegern Deutsch-Ostafrikas", *Korrespondenz-Blatt der Deutschen Gesellschaft für Anthropologie Ethnologie und Urgeschichte*. No. 49 (1918) 67.

Krelle, H. "Beiträge zur Kenntnis der Saramo-Religion", *Archiv für Anthropologie*, 23 (1935) 223-35.

Lambo, T.A. "Neuropsychiatric Observations in the Western Region of Nigeria", *British Medical Journal*, 2, (1956) 1388-94.

Marwick, M.G. "The Social Context of Cewa Witch Beliefs", *Africa*, Vol. 22, No. 3 (London: 1952) 215-233.

Raymond, W.D. "Native Materia Medica", *Tanganyika Notes and Records*, No. 2 (Dar es Salaam, 1936) 50-54.

Redmayne, Alison. "Hehe Medicine", *Tanganyika Notes and Records*, No. 70 (Dar es Salaam, July 1969) 29-40.

Siirala, Martti. "Our Changing Conception of Illness", *Journal of Religion and Health*, Vol. 4, No. 2 (1966) 105-118.

Swantz, Lloyd. "African Religions in Transition", Jyväskylä University, Summer Conference Papers (1969).

Swantz, Lloyd. "Health and Healing in Traditional African Thought and Practise in Tanzania", *Health and Healing*, Makumira Consultation, Evangelical Lutheran Church in Tanzania (Arusha, 1967).

Swantz, Marja-Liisa. "The Spirit Possession Cults and Their Social Setting in a Zaramo Coastal Community", Makerere Institute of Social Research (Kampala, 1967).

Swartz, Marc J. "Interpersonal Tensions, Modern Conditions, and Changes in the Frequency of Witchcraft/Sorcery Accusations", *African Urban Notes*, Vol. 4 (1969) 25-33.

Swartz, Marc J. "Inter-Communication Between the Urban and Rural Zaramo in the Dar es Salaam Area", Makerere Institute of Social Research (Kampala, 1967).

Swartz, Marc J. "Persistence and Adaptation of Some Traditional Institutions in an African City", Jyväskylä University, Summer Conference Papers (1969).

Swartz, Marc J. "The Zaramo of Dar es Salaam: a study of continuity and change", *Tanganyika Notes and Records*, No. 71 (Dar es Salaam, 1965) 154-164.

Swartz, Marc J. "Interpersonal Tensions, Modern Conditions, and Changes in the Frequency of Witchcraft/Sorcery Accusations", *African Urban Notes*, Vol. 4 (1969) 25-33.

Tanner, R.E.S. "Some Southern Province Trees With Their African Names and Uses", *Tanganyika Notes and Records*, No. 31 (1951) 61-70.

Weck, Dr. "Der Wahehe Arzt und Seine Wissenschaft", *Deutsches Kolonialblatt*, (1908) 1048-1051.

Unpublished Manuscripts

Chavanduka, G.L. "A Sociological Study of Illness and Health in an Urban African Community", Duplicated Manuscript No. 250, Dept. of Sociology, University College of Rhodesia (Salisbury, 1968).

Organization of African Unity, OAU Scientific Council for Africa, (duplicated document) L (65) 25 OAU/STRC, Lagos, 1965.

Organization of African Unity, OAU Scientific Council for Africa, (duplicated document) L (67) 12, OAU/STRC, Dakar, 1968.

Swantz, Marja-Liisa. "Some Aspects of the Life of the Zaramo", Dar es Salaam; Kibaha Nordic Project Community Health Seminar, 1967. (Duplicated manuscript)

Swantz, Marja-Liisa. "The Zaramo Woman in a Coastal Community", Dar es Salaam; Kibaha Nordic Project Community Health Seminar, 1967. (Duplicated manuscript).

Vermunt, Cornelius. "The Luguru", Morogoro, 1969 (Private manuscript).

Public Documents

Tanganyika Government. *The Laws of Tanganyika Territory*, Vols.I, II. London: Watmought Ltd., 1947.

Tanganyika Government Statistical Abstract, *"Africal Sample Census, 1957 "*, Dar es Salaam: Government Press, Statistical Abstracts 1966, 37.

Tanzania, United Republic of. *A Dar es Salaam Social Survey-1965*. Nairobi: Marco Surveys Ltd., 1968.